Tai Chi

for Better Breathing

Tai Chi

for Better Breathing

Relaxation exercises for asthma relief
and overall good health

Grandmaster
Gary Khor

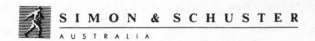
SIMON & SCHUSTER

AUSTRALIA

First published in Australia in 2001 by
Simon & Schuster (Australia) Pty Limited
20 Barcoo Street,
East Roseville NSW 2069

A Viacom Company
Sydney New York London Toronto Singapore

National Library of Australia
Cataloguing-in-Publication Data

Khor, Gary, 1947—
   Tai Chi for better breathing: relaxation exercises for
asthma relief and overall good health

   ISBN 0 7318 0996 3

   1. Asthma - Treatment. 2. Tai chi chuan - Therapeutic use.
   I. Title.

616.238062

Cover and text design: Greendot Design
Cover photograph: The Photo Library
Illustrator: Lorenzo Lucia
Set in Sabon 11pt on 14pt leading
Printed in Australia by Griffin Press

10 9 8 7 6 5 4 3 2 1

Contents

PART 3
The Body–Mind Exercise Session

The Body–Mind exercises

PART 4
Additional Body–Mind techniques for Asthma Management

BEFORE STARTING THE PROGRAM The advice given in this book is not intended as a substitute for advice from your medical practitioner. While all the exercises and techniques advised are generally safe for a person with asthma, your medical practitioner knows your specific medical condition and you should discuss this program with him/her before you begin.

REDUCTION OF MEDICATION It is, or should be, every asthmatic's aim to reduce their dependence on medication. The adoption of this program may well have the effect of improving your condition, thus allowing you to reduce your dependency on asthma-relieving drugs. However, any such action should only be taken in consultation with your medical practitioner. Reduction of medication without appropriate medical advice can be dangerous.

WHO SHOULD USE THIS BOOK The main aim of this book is to provide asthmatics with a Tai Chi-based exercise program that can help them manage and improve their condition. However, due to the holistic nature of Tai Chi, the practice of this program would also be of benefit those who have other breathing problems or who may be concerned that they are at risk of developing breathing problems such as asthma. Naturally those who are being treated for other breathing difficulties should always confer with their medical advisor as to the applicability of the exercises to their specific personal condition.

The program could also be used effectively to promote general health and/or as an introduction to Tai Chi-based exercise.

Foreword

Dr Michael Stanton graduated in medicine in England in 1967 and has been in full-time general practice in south-east Queensland, Australia, for the past 25 years.

Dr Stanton has studied many healing systems – naturopathy, herbalism, acupuncture, manual therapies and many aspects of Body–Mind medicine including relaxation, meditation and spiritual techniques.

Dr Stanton blends the best elements of these together with orthodox medicine to provide a holistic approach to diagnosis and treatment.

From the holistic perspective, asthma has two basic components:
* Tension;
* Stickiness, which causes spasm, phlegm, wheezing and coughing.

Tension can manifest itself in various ways. The significant body parts in asthma are the neck, throat, spine, diaphragm and muscles in the walls of the breathing tubes. Muscle tension can be alleviated by relaxation and exercise, and bronchial tension can be relaxed by avoiding irritants in the diet and environment as well as by relaxation techniques.

Stickiness occurs if normal body fluids become too thick. With asthma, sticky mucus clogs the airways, promoting spasm, cough and infection. Many years before asthma develops, stickiness may manifest as enlarged adenoids and tonsils with chronic mouth breathing and recurrent ear, nose and throat infections. Stickiness can be reduced by avoiding dietary and environmental irritants and by promoting exercise and deep breathing, which help prevent the accumulation of mucus.

Other factors in the development of asthma vary according to the individual and include genetic predisposition, type of infant feeding, digestive and bowel problems, and psychological factors.

In my early years of practice, I found it relatively easy to assist patients with general health exercises, diet, naturopathic treatments and counselling but having a busy practice didn't allow enough time to teach relaxation, meditation, breathing and postural exercise. I could only show the basics and then had to refer people off to a variety of other practitioners for health — physiotherapists, chiropractors, psychologists and counsellors. Patients found this exercise costly, fragmented and inefficient. I often wished for a 'one-stop shop' where people could learn all these things at the same time.

Then one early morning I was driving through Burleigh Heads on Queensland's Gold Coast and saw some people practicing slow, rhythmic movements in co-ordination. I was captivated by the calm graceful exercise and by the happy and relaxed appearance of the group. Making enquires I found that this exercise was Tai Chi. I immediately began to learn as much as I could about this wonderful art, as I could see its potential for healing as well as for relaxation and health maintenance.

I call Tai Chi the 'holistic exercise' because it exercises body, mind and spirit. The Chinese call it 'The Moving Meditation' and one cannot practice Tai Chi without automatically entering a more relaxed state of being. After some training, one can enter a deep meditative state during the exercise. The relaxed state energises the mind–body feedback loop and stimulates the immune system especially.

Tai Chi also exercises both halves of the body equally and thus, in contrast to many Western exercises and sports, stimulates the left and right hemispheres of the brain equally. The spiral, rotatory movements in Tai Chi are essential for good spinal posture and for healthy joints.

I was fortunate enough to make contact with the Australian Academy of Tai Chi in its early days and I learned Khor's Tai Chi with the Academy and enjoyed it immensely. I began recommending Tai Chi to patients with all sorts of problems and have since witnessed some extraordinary improvements in health due to Tai Chi. Over the past 20 years, many hundreds of my patients have reported improvement in their health problems after taking up the art, gaining general improvement in health, fitness and happiness.

I have noted Tai Chi to be of special benefit in treating arthritis, spinal problems, chronic fatigue, balance disorders, heart and blood pressure problems and, of course, chest conditions.

Asthma is especially amenable to improvement with Tai Chi because of the numerous interrelated effects the exercises have on the body and mind. Tai Chi promotes general fitness, vitality, and stimulates the immune system, all essential for basic good health.

Specifically, Tai Chi relaxes the neck and shoulder muscles, normalising upper torso posture, which in turn relaxes the throat and expands the chest. The rotatory movements relax the mid and lower spinal muscles, which in turn relaxes the lower rib cage and diaphragm, expanding the lower chest. The diaphragmatic movements also re-adjust the spinal posture as well as increase lung expansion. The empowerment of the breath prevents mucus and inhaled particles accumulating in the breathing tubes and the extra oxygen brought into the body helps burn up accumulated mucus as well as improving vitality. Improved oxygenation also enhances brain function, especially memory and concentration, which is often adversely effected by asthma.

The focus on breathing and co-ordinated calm, slow movements acts as an automatic meditation system promoting deep relaxation. After some practice, a conditioned reflex can be set up so that some asthmatics are able to learn to enter a relaxed state at the onset of an attack. Deep relaxation, together with diaphragmatic breathing, can often alleviate or even abort an attack of asthma. When the diaphragm moves correctly it massages and stimulates the abdominal and pelvic organs, helping to prevent digestive and bowel problems, which often exacerbate asthma.

Let me give a few examples of how Tai Chi helped some of my patients:

- First, there was a teenager I'll call Dan. He'd been asthmatic from infancy and did improve considerably when I changed his diet and gave him some naturopathic remedies. However, he was a very tense young man and it was hard to get him to relax. In sport, he favoured hard, contact sports that tended to increase his tension. I couldn't get him to relax enough to use his diaphragm. I suggested that he try Tai Chi, which he did and loved. After six months' practice, he was using his diaphragm efficiently, was a much more relaxed individual and was able to cease his residual medication. That was 15 years ago and as far as I know he remains cured of asthma.

- Another example involved a gentleman of about 50 years of age. He had a terrible chest, having been exposed to asbestos in the building industry as a youth when safety regulations were non-existent. Later in life he developed very severe chest disease, including asthma. After 12 months of Tai Chi, including some naturopathic treatments, his condition had improved so much that he was able to stop taking steroids on which he had been dependent for many years and his exercise tolerance was much improved.

- One woman had asthma associated with gross obesity. She had tried every diet and was on multiple drug therapy for the asthma. This lady diligently practiced her Tai Chi as part of a holistic treatment program and after six months her breathing had improved so much she was able to cease all prescription drugs. After a further year and a half, her body weight was normal and she considered herself rejuvenated by Tai Chi.

I have come to know Grandmaster Gary Khor very well over these past 20 years and consider myself fortunate to count him as a friend and colleague. Since its inception with a mere handful of students, Gary has led the Academy to great success in Australia and he now has the largest Tai Chi school outside of China. He has taught and inspired tens of thousands of Australians to achieve health, fitness and relaxation through Tai Chi and has also introduced us to many other ancient Chinese healing arts so that we may blend the best of Western medicine with the best of Chinese philosophy, culture and medicine.

Grandmaster Khor's latest book *Tai Chi for Better Breathing* is pertinent, concise, easy to read, and contains advice and suggestions invaluable to most asthmatics. It deserves a very wide readership and I wish Grandmaster Khor well in his work of promoting peace, health and happiness among us all.

DR MICHAEL STANTON

PART 1

Asthma and the Role of Body–Mind Medicine

Introduction

THE NUMBER OF PEOPLE with asthma in society is truly staggering and the incidence of asthma is still on the increase. Over the whole planet the quality of life of perhaps as many as half a billion people is being adversely affected. At this time there is no recognised 'cure' for asthma, although there are a number of techniques for 'managing' the condition. While there are a large number of sources of information about many of the asthma management techniques available, the subject of exercise, and particularly holistic exercise that uses body-mind medicine techniques, is one that is covered only lightly, if at all. Having had the opportunity within my own organisation (The Australian Academy of Tai Chi) to see the benefits that such exercises and techniques brought to instructors and students with asthma, I wanted to make the benefits of these techniques as widely available as possible. The development of the 'Body–Mind Medicine Program for Asthma Management' as detailed in this book is my attempt to achieve that objective. (For the sake of brevity I will in future refer to the program as the ABMM program.)

The ABMM program is designed so that it is suitable for both adults and children to practice. It is also set out in a manner that would allow medical practitioners to easily integrate the program into asthma management plans. While the ABMM program can be used independently, it is not intended to be used to replace other asthma management programs, for example, those primarily based on medication or diet. Rather it should be used to supplement such programs with a view to increasing the overall health, vitality and quality of life of those with asthma. In that the ABMM program adds to the selection of available techniques, it increases the chances of successful asthma management. In modern medical parlance it becomes part of a 'multi-modal management plan'.

> *The ABMM program is designed to be used in conjunction with directions from your medical practitioner and should be discussed with him or her prior to putting the program in practice.*

The aims of the ABMM program

The aims of the program are to raise the quality of life of those with asthma by:

- reducing the number of asthma attacks;
- reducing the severity of the attacks that do occur;
- reducing dependence on medication (see 'Medication note' at the end of this section);
- reducing the stress and tension associated with asthma;
- increasing the feeling of 'well-being' and combating feelings of depression and fatigue;
- increasing the opportunity to participate in sports, physical exercise and outdoor activities.

This is achieved by use of techniques that include the use of: posture, movement technique, breathing, self-acumassage, positive thinking skills and chi meditation. The central element of the ABMM program is a regular body-mind exercise schedule that incorporates the techniques listed above. The body-mind exercise schedule can be supplemented with additional techniques drawn from both traditional Chinese health approaches and the latest discoveries that have been made in the area of body-mind-medicine. All the ABMM program techniques approach the body from a holistic viewpoint but are specifically aimed at managing asthma through the strengthening of the body systems such as the respiratory and immune functions. The role of the mind and emotions is also taken into account with techniques that help to manage stress and encourage positive thinking.

You may wonder why this book goes to such lengths to explain how the various exercises and techniques impact on asthma, instead of simply detailing the exercises. The reason is that the whole point of body-mind-medicine is the recognition of the interplay between the mind, emotions and physical body. The more understanding you have of how the techniques work, the more confidence you will have in them. This confidence induces a positive state of mind that can have a real outcome on just how well these techniques work for you. You will therefore find that, in addition to presenting information on how the techniques are performed, there is also considerable information on the mechanics of asthma and how the various techniques act to modify the impacts of asthma, either directly or indirectly. Absorbing and understanding this material should be considered part of the ABMM program.

Children and the Asthma Management Program

The incidence of children with asthma is even higher than that of adults but whereas adults are (generally) responsible enough to carry out any necessary tasks associated with the successful management of asthma, children may be more resistant to undertaking such tasks. They may be particularly resistant to doing things that draw attention to their condition and make them feel different to other children.

This program has been designed so that adults and children can practise the program together. (While designed for those with asthma, because of its holistic basis, not only is the program safe for non-asthma sufferers to practice but they will discover significant health benefits from undertaking the exercise program.) There is in fact no need to emphasise to children that this is an asthma management program at all. The program can simply be presented as the family's 'keep-fit program'. All the exercises are well within the ability of a child to perform and the visualisations make them particularly useful for children.

What is asthma?

Asthma is far from a modern condition, with its existence having been recognised for thousands of years. The condition is identified by recurrent bouts of wheezing and coughing in which difficulty is found in getting adequate quantities of air into, and particularly out of, the lungs. The very word 'asthma' is derived from the ancient Greek meaning 'to pant or to breathe forcefully'.

The percentage of the population with asthma has increased significantly over the last few decades. However, despite the millions suffering from this condition and the length of time that asthma has been studied, the actual cause of the disease remains a matter of speculation and there is no known cure for the asthmatic condition itself. On the plus side we do have a good understanding of what takes place during an asthma attack and have a number of treatments for reducing both the frequency and severity of attacks.

Because there has never been any clear understanding of the initial causes of asthma, the preferred methods of treatment have often varied in accordance with whatever view of the 'likely cause' of asthma held sway at any particular point in time. Thus there have been a number of 'fashions' in the understanding and treatment of asthma. In the early part of the 20th century the conclusion was that asthma was a psychological condition. This was not a new belief as in the *Book of Asthma*, the first major writing on asthma back in 1190 by the physician Maimonides, psychological treatments had been recognised as being 'of great help'. As the 20th century progressed, the conviction that asthma was a 'conditioned' behavioural problem emerged. Later the view that it was an allergy condition became predominant.

Current thoughts are leaning towards it being 'genetic' in origin although breathing and dietary factors are also still being advanced as the cause of asthma.One fascinating sidelight that points to the difficulty in understanding the cause of asthma relates to multiple personalities within the same body. It has been noted that while some of the personalities may have quite severe asthma attacks, other personalities (in the same body!) do not experience asthma attacks even when deliberately exposed to the allergen that has been shown to initiate attacks in the other personalities residing in the same body. This does not mean that asthma is a mental rather than physical condition but it does show that the mental state can play a determining role in whether or not an asthma attack occurs in response to an asthma trigger even when the trigger is an allergic response.

Let us first look at asthma attacks. During an attack, the bronchi and bronchioles (the tubes within the lungs that carry the air between the trachea and alveoli, see diagram overleaf) become 'hyper-reactive' and contract in response to stimuli that would not affect a person who does not have asthma. There is also an increased production of mucus within the lungs, which further narrows the space available for the movement of air within the lung passageways.

The contraction of the airways is called 'broncho-spasm' or more commonly an 'asthma attack'. With the narrowing of the airways the quantity of air getting to the alveoli (the small sack-like structures of the lungs where oxygen passes into the blood stream and the carbon dioxide is eliminated) starts to fall. The changing levels of oxygen and carbon dioxide are registered by the body and the muscles that drive the breathing process are stimulated to work harder and faster. The only way that the body can speed up the movement of air is to lower the air pressure within the lungs on the in-breath to levels lower than normal and raise the air pressure within the lungs on the out-breath higher than would normally be the case.

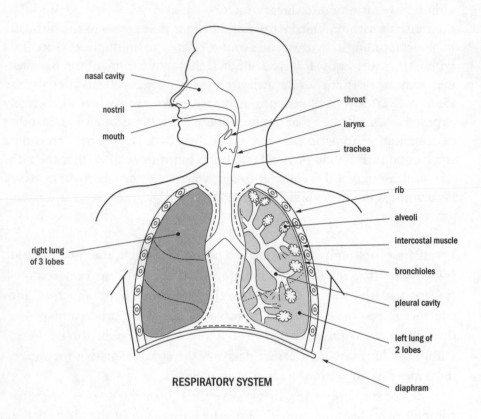

nasal cavity

nostril

mouth

throat

larynx

trachea

rib

alveoli

intercostal muscle

bronchioles

pleural cavity

right lung
of 3 lobes

left lung of
2 lobes

RESPIRATORY SYSTEM

diaphram

The fact that the breathing muscles must work much harder creates two important effects:

- First, the harder the breathing muscles work the more oxygen these muscles need to carry out their function. This means the lungs must take in yet more oxygen and the muscles must work yet harder again – a vicious cycle.
- Second, the harder the muscles work, the more a sensation of rigidity and tension is created within the body torso. A wheezing sound is created as the air rushes through the narrow passages. These sounds and sensations are noticed by the conscious mind, which then becomes aware that an asthma attack is developing. This

awareness naturally brings about anxiety. When the conscious mind becomes anxious, the breathing pattern starts to shift from longer deeper breaths to faster shallower breaths aggravating the effect of the asthma attack and creating another negative feedback cycle.

The narrowing of the air passages and the increased flow of mucus also increases the chance that the mucus lining on one side of the airway comes in contact with the mucus lining on the other side, causing a mucus plug to develop. This, and the higher air pressures and more rapid movement of air, can initiate coughing and further aggravate the attack. While virtually all asthma attacks pass without permanent injury to the asthma sufferer, a small number of attacks can spiral out of control and result in death. For this reason the management of asthma is always something that should be treated seriously.

The basic function of medication such as asthma inhalers is to disrupt the cascade of chemical effects which results in a full-blown asthma attack.

Triggers of asthma attacks

There are a number of 'triggers' to broncho-spasm or asthma attack. It is important that these triggers should not be seen as the cause of the asthma condition itself but only as the trigger for individual asthma attacks. However, while managing the triggers does not cure asthma, it does result in a much higher quality of life for the person with asthma. The reduction in the number of attacks also reduces the risks attached to asthma. The understanding and control of asthma triggers is thus a key element of asthma management.

It should also be realised that what may be a trigger for an asthma attack in one person may have no effect on another person with asthma. Whilst most people with asthma will find that they are subject to asthma attacks initiated by a number of triggers, a few will only be subject to one trigger and others again may need the simultaneous presence of a number of triggers before an asthma attack is initiated.

It is therefore important for asthma sufferers to determine exactly what triggers affect them. If you take asthma medication when you feel the onset of an asthma attack, then reducing or managing exposure to your triggers will lessen the number of potential attacks and also as a consequence the number of times you need to avail yourself of medication. The main types of triggers so far identified are:

- infection;
- allergy (pollen, dust mites, environmental pollutants, mould, spores, dust, smoke, food additives, animal products);
- stress and emotion;
- exertive exercise;
- abrupt temperature and humidity changes.

Let us look at these triggers individually.

INFECTION

Many of those with asthma find themselves more subject to attacks (or only subject to attacks) when they have colds, flu or similar infections. In such cases there is often either increased mucus that may block, or excessive coughing that may inflame, the airways within the lung. This additional stress on the lungs may tip the balance in favour of an asthma attack. Other factors associated with colds and flu that should not be forgotten are the increase in mental stress and depression that accompany such infections. Also, the immune system itself is under pressure. All these 'symptoms' of infection may themselves increase the vulnerability to asthma attack.

If colds and flu are acting as triggers to asthma attacks, then anything that reduces the chance of catching such infections will obviously help to manage asthma. While it may make sense to get the latest flu injection and avoid people with heavy colds, the fact is that flu injections only work against a particular strain of flu and you may only find out that someone has a cold when it is too late to prevent infection. Body–mind techniques that can reduce your chance of infection include:

- Keeping the immune system in tip-top condition;
- Controlling stress and negative emotion;
- Practising breathing techniques that minimise the chance of infection.

Techniques for achieving these objectives are included in the ABMM program.

ALLERGY

Attacks of asthma may be triggered when the presence of specific chemicals associated with such things as pollen, dust-mites, environmental pollutants, mould, spores, dust, smoke, food additives, animal products, etc come in contact with the surface of the lung membrane. Basically the body treats these substances in a similar way to invading microbes but the response is disproportionate, causing more damage than the substance itself would cause.

Two things are necessary for an allergic response: the presence of the allergen and a malfunction within the immune system. Whilst significant allergic attacks may sometimes result from very small amounts of allergen, most often there tends to be a critical level of exposure to the allergen which must be exceeded before the allergen results in a full-blown asthma attack. Thus, while it may not be possible to eliminate exposure to some allergens altogether, it may well be possible to keep this exposure below the critical level. The ABMM program looks at ways of strengthening the immune system, along with breathing techniques that reduce the quantity of matter that might trigger allergic substances getting into the lungs.

STRESS

There is plenty of evidence to show that stress and excessive emotion can play a major role in triggering asthma attack. The more that you can release stress, be relaxed and have a positive and optimistic approach to life, the more you will reduce your chances of having an asthma attack.

The role of stress in an asthma attack can be a vicious cycle as the stress and emotion generated by one asthma attack may then set up the conditions for the next asthma attack. Also the stress and emotion associated with one attack may increase the severity of that attack and thus the stress associated with that attack.

The movement, posture and breathing techniques detailed in the program not only relieve stress between asthma attacks but can be used to control stress during asthma attacks. The techniques also improve the feeling of well-being and the sense of mental vitality.

EXERCISE

When speaking of exercise as an 'asthma trigger', it is important to point out that there is a difference between 'exertive exercise' and the type of exercises included in the ABMM program, and that even exertive exercise of the most demanding kind does not necessarily trigger an asthma attack. There have been many outstanding athletes who have had asthma, including multiple Olympic Gold medal winner, Dawn Fraser.

It is obvious that one does not abandon eating or breathing because these may cause allergic response! Nor does one isolate oneself from contact with all other human beings because one may catch a cold from them. These would be gross overreactions that would put one in a much worse situation than having the asthma attack in the first place. In a like manner, one should not seek to avoid all challenge and exercise because the stress involved may trigger an asthma attack. While the negative consequences of avoiding exercise may not be as immediate as those of avoiding food, they are still serious and ultimately may be more life-threatening than an asthma attack. Rather, the secret lies in managing these factors and just as good diet, proper breathing and a rich and stimulating environment can be used to protect and strengthen the individual with asthma, the same is true for physical exercise.

To avoid physical exercise is to weaken the respiratory and immune systems, to increase the risk of depression and to contribute to a poor level of well-being. In fact, avoiding exercise may not prevent exercise-induced asthma attacks; it may simply lower the level of physical exercise required to bring on such an attack.

This is so because the main element of physical exercise that can stimulate an asthma attack is sudden, significant increases in the tidal volume of air being utilised by the body. Vigorous, sprint-type activities build up what is known as an 'oxygen debt'. That is, the muscles of the body use so much oxygen that the oxygen levels within the blood fall. This is a dangerous situation for the body – the brain and vital organs such as the heart cannot afford to stop because of a lack of adequate oxygen supplies. The body responds by speeding up the breathing process not only to meet current oxygen requirements but to rebuild the reservoir of oxygen within the blood. (This is why we continue to pant even after ceasing physical activity. If we continue to exercise, eventually we catch our 'second wind' as we repay the oxygen debt and only have to breathe to meet current oxygen requirements.) The greatest risk of asthma attack comes during the phase of exercise when breathing is fastest and the air is moving violently into and out of the lungs. That is during the oxygen payback period.

Lack of exercise tends to result in a situation where the smallest extra physical demand such as climbing stairs or making a sudden rush for a bus brings on an oxygen deficit and its associated panting period.

It is also during the 'payback' period that the volume of air required necessitates mouth rather than nose breathing. This means that the lungs are also exposed to unheated, unmoistened, unfiltered air, which raises the chance of drying out and irritation of the sensitive lung lining.

If we manage our exercise so that there is no oxygen debt and so that the volume of air required can be met by nasal breathing, then we can avoid the trigger effects of exercise. Slow, sustained exercise whose air requirements can be met through nasal breathing provide the solution. This is a particular feature of Tai Chi-based exercises and all exercises in this program meet these requirements. There is also the fact that these exercises are 'relaxing' rather than stressful.

It is most important that children do not begin to associate exercise with asthma (even if this is due to the well-intentioned warnings of carers). If they do, then they may become stressed and fearful each time that they find themselves in a situation where they are performing physical exercise. Then it may well become the case that it is the stress and fear associated with the exercise that becomes the asthma trigger, not the exercise itself. Involving children with asthma in an exercise program that can be performed without the risk of asthma attack can be a very positive experience for the child even aside from the physical benefits.

TEMPERATURE AND HUMIDITY CHANGE

The ability of abrupt changes in temperature and humidity to cause asthma attacks can be related to two factors: the potential effect on the delicate lung membrane and the level of stress being experienced by the body as a result of these changes. Again, appropriate breathing and stress management techniques may play a role in reducing the frequency and severity of asthma attacks.

Who is getting asthma?

In actual fact, we cannot answer this question and for all we know, if it turns out that asthma is genetically based, everyone could actually have the condition or genetic predisposition. On this basis it would seem that no-one is immune to the risk of asthma. It does not matter what your age or sex is. It does not matter where you live, in the country or city, in the developed or undeveloped world, there is still a significant risk that you will develop an asthmatic condition.

Indeed current predictions in Australia are that we will shortly be experiencing a level of one in four people developing asthma from childhood. Apart from the human cost in lost lives and degraded quality of life, there is a huge social cost in terms of lost productivity, absenteeism and creativity. The demand on medical resources and medication is enormous. Understanding and managing this condition therefore becomes most important.

There is statistical evidence that your likelihood of developing asthma is greater if the condition is present in your family history. However, a number of reasons have been put forward for this, as are discussed below.

Causes of asthma

As stated in the introduction, what the asthmatic condition is and how it is caused remains a matter for conjecture. This may sound incredible but the fact is that there is no physically detectable difference between the lungs of a person with asthma and the lungs of a person who does not have asthma. The only way you can tell whether someone has asthma or not is the presence of the asthma attacks themselves, including the early indications of such attacks, like changes in the tidal capacity of lungs.

The suspected causes of asthma include:
- genetic predisposition;
- allergic response;
- vitamin deficiency (vitamins A and B have been nominated);
- psychosomatic;
- incorrect breathing technique;

- mineral deficiency; and
- other dietary deficiency such as Omega 3 fatty acids.

While the adherents of each of these causes often have an almost religious zeal in proclaiming that theirs is the one and only one true cause of asthma, it appears much more likely that asthma is a complex disease that may have different causes in different people.

Looking at each of these potential causes can also tell us a little about the management approaches that may be effective with asthma.

GENETIC PREDISPOSITION

No 'genes for asthma' have been detected to date but the increased incidence of asthma in people who have a family history of asthma have led to speculation that such a gene, or group of genes, may exist. If it does, it is so variable in its operation that discovering it may do little other than add to our scientific knowledge. Many people whose parents have asthma fail to show any evidence of the condition. Also, in the opposite direction, many people develop asthma who have no family history of the disease. Of course it is possible to speculate that virtually everyone actually has the 'asthma gene' but that the gene is only 'turned on' under certain conditions. If we could identify an asthma gene, find out what turned on the gene, and then come up with a way of turning off the gene this would pave the way for the elimination of asthma. However, at this time we are not even at stage one, so while research in this area is potentially of vital importance to the long-term management of asthma, in the short to medium term we must look to other techniques.

It is noted in *Mind-Body Medicine*, edited by Daniel Coleman PhD, that with one asthmatic parent, children have a 20 per cent chance of developing the disease, whereas with two asthmatic parents this incidence increases to 50 per cent. Before the 'gene era' this was explained as either the children being 'conditioned' to develop asthma by concern over the asthma attacks of their parents or exposure to the same environment as had 'caused' the asthma in their parents. It could well be that all these factors contribute to the expression of asthma as asthma attacks.

We should also be aware of the fact that just because a particular gene may 'predispose' us to a condition, it does not mean that that condition cannot arise from other causes as well. In this regard the reader may recall that there is both a genetic predisposition to diabetes and diabetes resulting from failure or damage to the pancreatic function.

ALLERGIC RESPONSE
We know that many asthma attacks are initiated by allergic responses to a large variety of substances and that the very nature of broncho-spasm is that of an out of control immune response. Supporters of the 'allergy school' believe that something causes the respiratory system to become 'sensitised' to various substances encountered through diet, touch or inhalation. If allergic response is the cause of asthma as well as the trigger for subsequent attacks, it does little to explain the success of many of the management techniques that reduce the incidence of asthma attacks.

VITAMIN DEFICIENCY (VITAMINS A AND B HAVE BEEN NOMINATED)
The proposal that vitamin deficiency is the cause of asthma is put forward because of the success in reducing the incidence of asthma attacks in some asthmatics when the quantity of these vitamins in the diet is increased. (But see notes on dangers of excessive levels of vitamin A.) It is conjectured that a shortage of vitamins A and B may be involved in the defective immune response to allergens. Vitamin C is also useful in reducing asthma attacks related to infection triggers because of its effect in enhancing the immune response rather than any direct effect on asthma.

PSYCHOSOMATIC
Back in the early part of the 20th century, prevailing medical opinion was that asthma was a psychological condition, a form of hysteria resulting from deep anxiety. Later, with the rise of the 'behaviourist school', it was thought that children who witnessed this condition in their parents or close family members had become 'conditioned' to develop the problem themselves. It is now felt that while psychological factors play an important role in the frequency and severity of attacks, they are not involved in the development of the condition itself.

INCORRECT BREATHING TECHNIQUE
This is a relatively modern concept attributed to Professor Butyenko, that asthma is developed in response to persistent 'overbreathing'.

Breath training seems to have considerable impact on reducing the frequency and severity of asthma attacks. It would also go some way to explaining family clusters of asthma sufferers since parents' breathing routines are often subconsciously adopted by their children. Again, while the importance of proper breathing technique to the management and control of asthma should not be underestimated, assuming asthma is solely due to breathing problems does little to explain the success of other asthma management techniques.

MINERAL AND OTHER DIETARY DEFICIENCIES (OMEGA 3 FATTY ACIDS)

Some asthmatics show a marked decrease in asthma attacks on being given mineral supplements or omega 3 fatty acids. Again, the conjecture is that a shortage of these substances is interfering with the immune response. Once more, there may be no direct effect on asthma other than that derived from a better state of general health but it would seem silly not to try anything that may make you healthier and reduce the instance of asthma attacks.

The Body–Mind Medicine Perspective on Asthma

The body–mind medicine perspective acknowledges that the mind can often play a decisive role in healing. Ask any doctor how much harder their job is if the patient has little or no will to get better. How does the mind influence the body? How far can this influence go? These are subjects of intense investigation with many practitioners in the area defining the boundaries and possibilities of the field differently. When I speak of body-mind-medicine, I am using the term in the traditional Chinese context. (So far all the latest research and development that I have seen in body–mind medicine can be accommodated within the traditional Chinese concepts.)

Long ago the Chinese came up with a concept for how the mind and body influenced each other by seeing the world as various flows and interactions of *chi* (or life energy). In traditional Chinese medical terms, all disease is the result of disruption to the proper flow of *chi*. From a Chinese perspective, diseases are thus just 'symptoms' and the proper thing to do is to correct the energy flow. Techniques such as acupuncture, acupressure, moxibustion, *chi kung* exercises, *chi* breathing, *chi* meditation and *chi* diet are all designed to balance and harmonise the flow of *chi* energy. To the Chinese, all healing is body-mind-medicine because there is always the consideration of how the *chi* associated with the mind and emotion of both the patient and healer is influencing the rebalancing of energy or *chi*.

To reiterate, from a Chinese perspective, asthma is the consequence of an energy imbalance or blockage. This imbalance can be corrected by any technique that encourages energy to flow correctly. In all these techniques the state and focus of the mind plays an important role. The ABMM program techniques are drawn from the traditional Chinese healing techniques mentioned above, excluding acupuncture (and this only because appropriate training is necessary to avoid risk of injury or incorrect application).

The traditional Chinese approach also recognises the 'body-mind' connection in a way that the West is still coming to terms with. If you say to a Western person that their condition is 'psychosomatic', they will tend to feel insulted as the idea that the body's problem is caused by the mind is interpreted as either saying that their problem is in some way 'unreal' or their 'fault'.

To the Chinese, the energy of the mind and the emotions is no more and no less real than the energy of the body and just as capable of causing or healing disease. To get the energy balance corrected, as much attention is paid to the mind as is paid to the body. To demonstrate the point, it has been shown that if your asthma attacks are triggered by allergic responses, say to a cat or flower, then simply seeing the cat or flower can trigger an asthma attack – even if the cat or flower are being viewed through glass. Even more amazingly, some people who are allergic to roses have had an attack by being presented with artificial substitutes such as plastic and paper roses even though they are well aware that these are not 'real'.

This link of mind and body has been a thorn in the side of Western scientists for a long time. The placebo effect, in which the patient recovers simply because he believes that the cure he has been given should work, despite the fact that the cure has no real value whatsoever, has been the reason for the design of torturous and expensive 'double blind' experiments. In these experiments neither the recipient nor the experimenter must know which are the real cures and which are placebo cures being given, as this 'knowledge' has been shown to effect the outcome. You might think that the reason the experimenter must not know the real and placebo cures is because in some way he will communicate this knowledge to the patient, who will then have a different 'belief' about the cure and whether it will work and it is this belief that drives the body's physical response. In fact the situation may be even stranger than this.

Recent experiments at Stanford University to measure relaxation responses through biofeedback use showed that even if only one subject used a biofeedback technique, another subject nearby would also relax at the same time, even though they could not see or hear the subject using the biofeedback technique and had no idea when the technique was being used. In other words the subjects were somehow 'sensitised' by non-visual, non-verbal means to each other's state of relaxation or state of mind! We end up with a situation where not only the patient's expectation of success but the experimenters can affect the real outcome. Therefore we should not be surprised if a person administering a program of Vitamin A who believes that this will work experiences positive results, while a block away another person who believes that proper breathing techniques will reduce the incidence and severity of asthma attacks is also finding success.

The problem is not that we can reduce the frequency and severity of asthma attacks in different ways, but that we may not try anything until we are satisfied that it is the 'one and only cure'. For all we know the mind may be the 'one and only cure' and everything else we do is simply to convince the mind of the patient and/or the mind of the caregiver that a cure will be effected!

The approach taken in this program is that it is simply common sense to do whatever we can to improve the health of both the body and mind to help manage asthma. Sometimes there may be an obvious connection to the actual asthma attack, such as learning to apply breathing techniques that protect and maintain the health of lung tissue. Other times they will be more indirect, such as lessen the stress levels of the body. Reductions in stress levels do not only lessen the risk of stress-induced asthma attacks but they also have a positive effect on the immune system. When the immune system is operating well, there is less chance of it going off the rails and allowing the body to become sensitised to allergens, and more chance of preventing colds and infections that may contribute to the frequency and severity of asthma attacks.

Note You will find the term Tai Chi used quite frequently. This is not only because various exercises and techniques are drawn from the practice of Tai Chi but because Tai Chi involves a whole philosophy of approach involving the balancing of individuals at all levels – physically, mentally and emotionally. Achieving such a balance is not only a good way to manage asthma but a good way to manage one's life.

Using this book

The structure of this book recognises that people have different approaches to the way they take on any new activity. Some like to dive straight into the activity itself, perhaps later returning to build up their understanding of the theory of what they are doing. Others like to absorb the theory first, then perform the activity. Others again simply have a few key questions they want answered before they put their time into theory or practice. This book caters for all these different approaches.

- Those who simply want to 'dive in and do' should proceed directly to Parts 3 and 4 of the book.
- Those who want certain key questions answered first should start at Part 2.
- Those who want to understand the theory as well as the practice should look at both Parts 2 and 3 before commencing the program.

The book includes basic explanations of the way that the exercises function in respect of asthma, both from Western and Chinese perspectives. Please recognise, however, that this is not a medical text and it is beyond the scope of this book to deal with the medical theory underlying the exercises at any great depth. For those interested in extending their knowledge further than the material outlined in this book, included in the appendices are a list of other books and publications, available from the AATC, on such matters as relaxation theory, *chi* theory, breathing and meditation, nutrition, acupressure and massage etc.

For those with 'key questions', obviously we cannot cover all the questions you might have and have included only the most common questions asked about Tai Chi and asthma. If you have other questions (as long as they don't relate to medical advice — your medical practitioner is your best source there), we can be contacted by post, email, phone and fax at the contact details provided in the appendices.

Important note about medication

Whilst I know from my own experience of instructors and students with asthma who have been able to significantly reduce or even dispense with medication after taking up the regular performance of the exercises and techniques outlined in this book, I cannot stress strongly enough that the levels of medication were reduced on the advice of medical practitioners after it was found that they were no longer needed. Any reduction of medication prior to your medical practitioners' advice that it is no longer needed can be very dangerous and even life-threatening. Nothing that you read in this book should be construed as supporting that you personally reduce your medication or the medication of anyone within your care.

This book does not contain any advice on drug-based medication because there are a number of such books already available by other persons with more detailed knowledge and qualifications in that area. Also consider that your medical practitioners is more likely to be up to date with the latest information on these subjects.

PART 2

How The Asthma Body–Mind Medicine Program Works

THIS PART OF THE BOOK has two objectives. First, I want to leave you without any excuses for you not giving the ABMM program a try! Once you do, I am sure that you will stay with it. Of course I recognise that some people will have concerns that need to be addressed before they will be comfortable trying the ABMM program. The first section of Part 2 is therefore a collection of the most commonly asked questions about the ABMM program – along with my response. Second, as previously noted in Part 1, the body-mind element of the ABMM program is not just hype to make the program, look good, it's real and it has real consequences. That means that the more confidence you have in the ABMM program the better the results will be for you. To provide this confidence, the second section of Part 2 explains the 'how and why' of the ABMM program.

If you are somebody who likes to 'get in and do', or you do not have any particular concerns about trying out the ABMM program and you are not particularly theory-orientated, then you can proceed directly to Part 3 of this book and leave the theory aside until some more appropriate time for you.

Questions and Answers about Asthma and the ABMM Program

1. ARE ABMM PROGRAM EXERCISES 'SAFE' FOR ASTHMATICS? WHY?

The concern here is generally related to the risk of the exercise acting as a 'trigger' for an asthma attack. In 'Triggers of asthma attacks' (page 9), it was discussed how one had to distinguish between 'exertive' and 'non-exertive' exercise with the former being the cause of exercise-triggered asthma attacks.

Since ABMM program exercises are 'non-exertive in nature', the general answer to the question of safety is that, yes, the exercises are safe. However, there can always be individual factors to consider and you should discuss your participation in this (or any other) program with your medical practitioner.

The reason that ABMM program exercises are the safest form of exercise for those with asthma is because they have the following features:

- **The exercises are performed in a relaxed state.** This is important for those with asthma because when the body becomes stressed, not only do muscles surrounding the chest area become tighter (making it more difficult to breathe) but the breath rate tends to be faster and shallower than it should be. Competitive exercise (while fun) tends to increase stress levels and impact on breathing.
- **The exercises are performed with good posture.** The emphasis on the straight, vertical spine maximises the natural lung capacity, allowing the breath rate to be slower.
- **The exercises do not build up an 'oxygen debt' (see page 12).** Avoiding oxygen debt avoids the excessively forceful breathing associated with the 'payback' period and makes it easier to maintain nasal breathing.
- **The exercises focus on nasal breathing.** This makes sure that the air taken into the lungs is properly filtered, moistened and at the right temperature and thus less likely to aggravate sensitive lung tissue.
- **The exercises focus on the use of a natural, unforced diaphragmatic breathing.** The emphasis is on keeping the breath quiet and smooth, and avoiding forced excessive intake of air sometimes referred to as overbreathing or hyperventilation. As such, the breathing techniques used in the ABMM program are particularly suitable for asthmatics.

2. DO THE BENEFITS THAT ABMM PROGRAM EXERCISES HAVE FOR ASTHMA DEPEND ON THE CAUSE OF THE ASTHMA?

Essentially the concern here is that if the cause of the asthma is due to such things as allergic response, genetic predisposition, emotional state etc, will there be any benefit from carrying out a predominantly exercise-based program?

The answer to this is that the ABMM program exercises may work in various ways, depending on the original cause of the asthmatic condition, but the benefits derived will remain. To understand why this is so, let us review what we discussed about the potential causes of asthma and asthma attacks in Part 1 and see how ABMM program exercises could benefit those with asthma. It should be remembered that what we are looking at here is the potential cause of the asthmatic condition, not the trigger for attacks. (To complicate matters some of the suggested causes are also known to act as triggers.)

Note Only the general nature of the benefits of the ABMM program exercises on asthma is described in the answer to this question. A more detailed analysis of the mechanisms by which the benefits are delivered follows in the next section 'The How and Why of ABMM'.

ASTHMA AS AN ALLERGIC REACTION

We do not have a complete explanation of why the body, often quite suddenly, becomes sensitised to certain substances. There is, however, substantial evidence that suggests that a run-down immunological system may be involved in such sensitisation. ABMM Program exercises can work on a number of levels, such as:

- improving the immune system itself;
- reducing the amount of work that the immune system has to perform;
- reducing exposure to the irritants that may trigger an allergic asthmatic response.

Stress has a significant adverse impact on the immune system. ABMM program exercises help increase the ratio of the time the body spends in relaxation response as compared to stress response. With its holistic approach, ABMM program exercises strengthen the respiratory function. Further, correct breathing techniques can both reduce the volume of muck that gets into the lungs and the effect of environmental stresses (such as those caused by cold and dry air) on the sensitive lung lining.

ASTHMA AS A DIETARY DEFICIENCY

This theory normally identifies the cause of asthma as a result of a shortage of vitamin A or B (sometimes magnesium deficiency or lack of omega 3 fatty acids are identified as the cause). What is suggested here is that dietary deficiency causes problems in lung function either directly or because of impact on body systems that support the lung function. If the asthma is caused directly by a dietary deficiency, then obviously identification and rectification of the dietary deficiency should be the main objective. However, if the dietary deficiency results in asthma because of impact on body systems, then the ABMM program exercise has a role to play in supporting the lung function. This becomes even more important if the deficiency-related problem was due to vitamin A. This is because large quantities of vitamin A can have a number of serious adverse side-effects. In other words, the healthier the lung function, the lower the quantities of such vitamin supplements will need to be.

Also, dietary deficiency can be as much a result of problems with your digestive process as your base diet. There is not much point in taking expensive vitamin supplements if these simply pass directly through the alimentary tract without being absorbed by the body. The ABMM program exercises work to improve the digestive function both through its internal massaging effect and the reduction of stress in the body, which can improve blood supply and circulation to the digestive organs. There is also some suggestion that stress acts to disturb the balance of the micro-organisms found along the intestinal tract, which again impacts adversely on balanced digestion. The reduction in stress levels from the ABMM program will assist in the maintenance of this balance.

> *Nothing in this section or elsewhere in the book should be read as a recommendation that you should start taking vitamin A supplements, although I do suggest that you look at your diet to ensure that it is properly balanced and does contain the recommended intake of natural vitamin A. The decision to take vitamin A supplements is best discussed with your medical practitioner.*

ASTHMA AS A BREATHING PROBLEM (LEARNED OR GENETIC)

There are some recent suggestions that the cause of asthma may be sourced to poor breathing practices such as:

- hyperventilation (taking in more air over a given period of time than is required to meet the body's needs); and
- breathing through the mouth (which exposes the lungs to environmental stress and substantial increased exposure to infection.

The ABMM program exercises teach good breathing habits, including nasal breathing and a easy approach to breathing where the breath is easy and unforced. Again the holistic impact of improving the lung function, the reduction of stress and the strengthening of the immunological system can only improve matters for the asthmatic.

You may have heard of the Butyenko breathing method, which claims great success in treating asthma. One sometimes hears that this states deep breathing is bad but in fact what Professor Butyenko says is that 'over-breathing' is bad, which is quite different to deep breathing. Actually Professor Butyenko's book recommends Tai Chi and its associated breathing techniques.

Whatever the cause, or combination of causes, of the source of the asthmatic condition turns out to be, ABMM program exercises have considerable benefits to offer.

3. WHAT BENEFITS CAN ONE EXPECT FROM THE PHYSICAL EXERCISE ASPECT OF ABMM PROGRAM EXERCISES?

The benefits fall into two specific areas. Firstly, the general benefits that any practitioner of the Tai Chi-based exercises used in the ABMM program could expect to receive and secondly, those benefits that are specific to asthma sufferers.

GENERAL BENEFITS OF ABMM PROGRAM EXERCISES

The general health benefits derived from the practice of the Tai Chi-based ABMM program exercises should not be overlooked by those focused on specific health problems. People from all ages and walks of life take up Tai Chi-based exercise for the health and quality of life benefits it brings (not to mention the fact that it is an enjoyable and fascinating activity in its own right).

For centuries Tai Chi has had a reputation as a health-building exercise system. Modern research has confirmed this and revealed the art as a particularly sophisticated health system. Many other exercise systems limit their focus to development of the cardiovascular, muscular and respiratory systems, whereas Tai Chi is holistic and equally focused on all the major body systems including:

* the health of the internal organs such as heart, lungs, liver, kidneys, spleen and pancreas;

- the endocrine and immunological systems;
- posture and the health of the spine;
- joints and co-ordination;
- digestion;
- mental functions. It promotes a positive and optimistic approach to life, helping to overcome depression.

Tai Chi is also an excellent stress management system. (If the reader wants a more detailed explanation of all the general benefits of Tai Chi and the mechanisms by which these benefits are brought, they are referred to other AATC publications as are detailed in the appendices of this book.)

SPECIFIC BENEFITS OF ABMM PROGRAM EXERCISES FOR THOSE WITH ASTHMA

These are:
- improvement of the health of the lungs and respiratory system;
- reduction in the chance of the infection of the lungs;
- breathing techniques that help reduce the likelihood of asthmatic attacks from triggers such as allergens, stress, exercise, temperature and moisture changes;
- breathing techniques that can reduce the severity and impact of asthmatic effects;
- benefits that can partially offset negative consequences created by an asthmatic condition (tendency to depression and lack of vitality);
- increased efficiency in the digestive process that may assist in the uptake of micronutrients that may play a role in the asthmatic condition and that will improve the overall health of the body.

The detailed theory behind each of these specific benefits is explained in the answer to question 7 in this section.

4. ARE THERE SPECIAL RISKS ATTACHED TO THE ABMM PROGRAM FOR CHILDREN WITH ASTHMA?

The answer to this question is that while there are fewer risks attached to the ABMM program exercises than many other physical activities that children undertake, studies have shown that the proportion of exercise-triggered asthma attacks in children is higher than that in adults. It is quite possible that this increased proportion of exercise-induced attacks simply reflects the fact that children act like children and therefore tend to participate more frequently in strenuous exercise than the average adult asthma sufferer does. The increased proportion of exercise-induced attacks may also reflect the fact that children are less mature in their judgement of when enough exercise is 'enough'.

The fact is that the nature of children means that they will be exposed to more risk of exercise-induced asthma attacks. The strenuous exercise, the rushing around, the environmental changes (as they fly in and out of the house a hundred times a day) all increase the risk of an attack. To teach children to fear these things would be a totally negative approach that would severely damage the child's quality of life. There is also the risk that if children become stressed about the risk of exercise, then one may be creating a self-fulfilling prophecy, where it is the stress of worry over the exercise that triggers the attack rather than the exercise itself.

5. ARE THERE ANY SPECIAL BENEFITS OF THE ABMM PROGRAM FOR CHILDREN WITH ASTHMA?

ASSISTANCE WITH SCHOOL WORK AND EXAMS

It may seem strange to claim that participation in Tai Chi-based exercise programs may have a beneficial effect on school work but some schools (primary and secondary) have included AATC exercise programs as part of their curriculum. Not only do children appear to enjoy them but there are reports that there is a general improvement in the ability to focus and concentrate.

In essence, as a body-mind exercise, Tai Chi-based exercise improves the ability to focus and concentrate for extended periods of time. Once a child has gained this ability, it is not limited to exercise but may be used in any activity in life including school work! Also not to be underestimated is the fact that Tai Chi-based exercise improves health and creates a more positive mindset. This will be of assistance in understanding and memorising learning material.

Not only can Tai Chi-based exercise assist in making sure that a child is better prepared intellectually for an exam, but the breathing and relaxation techniques can be of value in overcoming the stress and anxiety that often accompanies exams. With the significance that stress has for people with asthma, any reduction in stress particularly at exam times, can be of particular value. Probably the worst time for a child to have an asthma attack is before or in the middle of an exam!

ASSISTANCE WITH SPORTING ACTIVITIES AND PHYSICAL GAMES

As noted above with children being what they are, they will frequently engage in organised sports and 'disorganised' physical games. The breathing techniques that Tai Chi-based exercises teach will assist in protecting the lungs. The relaxation techniques will help reduce any stress involved in competitive sport. The increased general level of health and co-ordination will also assist at a performance level.

6. HOW DO CHILDREN RESPOND TO THE EXERCISES IN THE ABMM PROGRAM?

The concern here may arise out of what people have heard about children's response to learning the Tai Chi form and whether there will be a similar response to the Tai Chi-based exercises found in the ABMM program.

In general it has been found that few children respond positively to learning the Tai Chi form in mixed classes of adults and children. The slowness of the movements, the focus on relaxation, the necessity to focus and concentrate, the two-year time frame involved in learning a connected sequence of 108 movements are generally unappealing to most children. These difficulties have long been recognised by the Academy and considerable work and experimentation has taken place to find out how these problems can be overcome so that children can benefit from Tai Chi.

Several exercise programs run at primary and high schools showed that children could not only respond positively but enthusiastically to learning the Tai Chi form when this was presented at a children's level, rather than an adult level. It was also discovered that if, instead of teaching the traditional form, one taught movements that used the same Tai Chi principles but that were repeated several times over, then children found the movements easier and more enjoyable to learn. (This was also found to be true for many adults.) This is the structure that has been used in the ABMM program.

Not only is the focus of the ABMM program on more simple exercise but on exercises that have much more visualisation associated with them than is usually found in learning the Tai Chi form. Children respond well to imagery and this leads to a much better body-mind connection and consequently more benefit. Adults tend to have the opposite focus to children; they can become almost obsessive about the structure of movements and are often most reluctant to use their imagination and visualisation, so these techniques can benefit adults too.

For children who wish to extend their exercises beyond those in this program, a special program has been developed along with video, and this is available from the Academy.

7. HOW ARE THE SPECIFIC ABMM PROGRAM HEALTH BENEFITS FOR ASTHMATICS ACHIEVED?

The specific ABMM program benefits that we will look at in detail are:

- improvement of the health of the lungs and respiratory system;
- reduction in the risk of infection of the lungs;
- breathing techniques that help reduce the likelihood of asthmatic attacks from triggers such as allergens, stress, exercise, temperature and moisture changes;
- breathing techniques that can reduce the severity and impact of asthmatic effects;
- benefits that can partially offset negative consequences created by an asthmatic condition (tendency to depression and lack of vitality);
- improvement in the digestive process, which will assist in the uptake of micronutrients that may play a role in the asthmatic condition, and will improve the overall health of the body.

IMPROVEMENT OF THE HEALTH OF THE LUNGS AND RESPIRATORY SYSTEM

While the theory behind the benefits of Tai Chi breathing techniques has been explained above, it is also important to remember that while the mechanisms of Tai Chi are entirely consistent with the Western understanding of the way the body functions, the techniques were actually derived from the Chinese understanding of body function.

A brief review of this understanding can shed some additional perspective on how Tai Chi breathing works.

It has been noted (see Part 1) that from the Chinese perspective, all sickness and illness is the result of irregularities in the flow of *chi* or 'life energy'. If the *chi* energy is excessive or deficient, or is not of the proper quality, then the result will be illness. *Chi* energy underlies the functioning of all the organs, including the lungs.

Chi is distributed throughout the body along a system of organ meridians known as the '*ching lo*'. If you think of these as like the magnetic lines of force that surround and permeate a magnet, you will have a usable working concept. Blockages in the flow of energy along the meridian impacts directly on the health of the organ function that is associated with the meridian. There are, however, a number of simple techniques for removing these blockages and ensuring that the *chi* flows freely along the meridian. Tai Chi has positive effects on *chi* flow through the following mechanisms:

- The elimination of constrictions on energy flow in the meridian caused by stress-induced muscular tension or poor posture.
- The encouragement of the flow of *chi* energy through:
  – sound movement techniques;
  – the internal massaging effects of Tai Chi;
  – visualisation techniques used in Tai Chi.

Strong *chi* in the lung meridian will not only improve lung functionality but also help protect against lung infections and disease. From a Western medical viewpoint, the sound breathing techniques taught will help to ensure that the lungs are not unduly stressed.

Diet, lifestyle and environment all play a role in the level of health of the lungs. Tai Chi principles have far wider application than just exercise. Applying Tai Chi principles to these other areas such as acupressure, massage and moxibustion can provide simple and easy-to-use techniques that can help maintain and improve lung function.

REDUCTION IN THE RISK OF THE INFECTION AND DISEASE OF THE LUNGS

Taking air into the lungs is one of those activities that, while necessary to sustain life, carries with it considerable risk. Along with the life-giving air come all sorts of bacteria, viruses and other agents that may cause disease and infection. Even worse, because these diseases are airborne, they often utilise the lungs of the person they have infected to spread themselves to the next victim. Thus we find ourselves coughing, sneezing and spluttering, our lungs and airways full of mucus and other discharge. While this serves the germ's need to spread itself to other victims, it generally results in increased lung dysfunction and inefficiency. This may be annoying if you have no other health problems, but for asthma sufferers it can create real problems. Anything that we can do to minimise the risk of disease and infection within the lungs is important.

It is self-evident that the less bacteria and viruses that get into the lungs, the lower the risk of lung infection will be. Nature has equipped us with a very effective piece of filtering equipment – the nose. One could suspect that many people would look at the size of the nostril and feel that it's not going to be much use in filtering out something as small as a virus or bacterium. But this is wrong. The nose is not designed to work like filter paper; rather, it is designed to create turbulent streams of air. These currents of air virtually guarantee that all of the air inhaled is brought into close contact with nasal tissue. This tissue is damp and moist, and designed so that the unwanted agents inhaled with the air stick to it and are then removed by mucus discharge. Thus the lungs and airways will have a greatly reduced infectious load with which to deal. The secondary defences within the lungs will thus be less likely to be overwhelmed by airborne diseases.

The filtering process is not limited to within the nose. The trachea and major bronchi have their walls covered in mucus, which is continually flowing upward to expel all of the various germs and irritants that get caught in its sticky embrace. When you breathe through the mouth, these airways dry out and their defensive capability is greatly reduced.

The nose also acts to reduce the chance of infection in another way. Infection is best fought off if the lung tissue is healthy. While, as discussed above, such health is primarily dependent on the underlying health of the lung function, it should also be appreciated that the lungs are designed to work on warm, moist air. If you breathe in through the nose then the air will arrive at the lungs moistened and heated. If you gulp air in through the mouth, then the air may be dry and cold. Dry air dries out the moist surfaces of the lungs. This makes them easier to infect. Cold air lowers the temperature of the lung lining, inhibiting many of the chemical reactions and reducing the effectiveness of any immune response.

Learning to breathe through your nose is a vital part of protecting yourself against infection. We shall also see in other sections that nasal breathing has many other advantages and benefits. A question might arise in your mind as to why, if nasal breathing is so advantageous, we ever evolved the ability to breathe through the mouth as well. There are two reasons for this:

1. The nasal passages are much narrower than the mouth and thus more vulnerable to being blocked. It makes good evolutionary sense to have a back-up system.
2. The body sometimes faces critical situations in which it is important that the body act with as much speed and strength as possible. The metabolic activity required to support such action requires much greater quantities of oxygen than normal. The nose cannot always deliver sufficient quantities of air in the time period required and therefore we have developed a mechanism where we can gulp in through the mouth the vast quantities of air required.

This is another version of the short-term/long-term health trade-off that we spoke about when discussing the stress response. Why worry about the risk of infection to the lungs when the major concern is to get the body out the way of that oncoming truck?

All this has some implication for strenuous exercise, which by its very nature, requires us to shift from nose to mouth breathing. Nature never envisaged performing any strenuous activity that did not have survival benefits (for the genes if not the body!). If our focus is on the body's long-term survival, then non-strenuous exercises such as Tai Chi, which do not force one into mouth breathing, are healthier. That is not to say that strenuous exercises cannot be fun-filled and stimulating, just that we should not operate under the illusion that it is the best way to health. This observation is particularly relevant to those suffering breathing disorders.

On a lighter note, if you are focused on the survival of your genes rather than your body, then strenuous exercise is recommended, since its results, in terms of body appearance, generally have a much greater attraction for the opposite sex! When one looks at the continued preference for strenuous exercise over gentle exercise, particularly in the younger post-puberty period, you could well believe that Professor Dawkins (author of *The Selfish Gene*) is right in suggesting that our bodies are gene-carrying vehicles that will tend to act in the long-term interests of the genes — not the human being carrying them! So why not reassert a little authority over your genes and practice gentle exercise?

Again, if we look at the Chinese perspective we should see the body's defensive systems on an energetic as well as physical level. The name given to this defensive energy is *wei chi* (literally external *chi)*. Strong *wei chi* acts as a barrier against infection and disease. The strength of *wei chi* is dependent on the strength of the *chi* within the body as a whole.

There are strong parallels here to the Western viewpoint, where we accept that the resistance of the lungs to disease and infection is dependent on an immune system, which in turn is influenced by the overall health of the body. The main difference is that the East looks at the situation from the viewpoint of energies and the West looks at it from the point of view of physical components and molecular reactions.

REDUCTION IN RISK OF ASTHMATIC ATTACKS FROM TRIGGERS SUCH AS ALLERGENS, STRESS, EXERCISE, TEMPERATURE AND MOISTURE CHANGES

We have discussed the reduction in the chances of infection that occur when you breathe through the nose, resulting in air that is properly warmed, moistened and filtered. These very same processes can help reduce exposures to asthma attack triggers.

Where asthma attacks are triggered by airborne allergens to which lung tissue is sensitised (such as pollens), then nose breathing stands a good chance of filtering out sufficient quantities of the allergen to either prevent an attack or at least substantially reduce it.

It is also known that cold dry air and particularly abrupt changes to cold dry air can trigger asthma attacks. Nose breathing will help to protect against these.

REDUCTION IN THE SEVERITY AND IMPACT OF ASTHMATIC ATTACKS

Whatever the initial cause of an asthma attack, the physical, emotional and psychological stresses that are associated with such an attack can make a bad situation worse. In effect, an asthma attack causes stress symptoms that makes the asthma attack worse. This then makes the attack victim more stressed, creating a vicious cycle. To the degree that these symptoms can be controlled, the impact and severity of asthma attacks will be reduced.

Let it again be emphasised – first follow the instructions that your medical practitioner has given you regarding medication etc. Then follow the ABMM exercise techniques in so far as they do not conflict with any previous medical advice.

In an asthmatic attack the natural tendency is to try to gulp large quantities of air as quickly as possible. Unfortunately quick shallow breathing acts to raise anxiety levels. The body responds by raising metabolic activity, which requires more oxygen, then the body struggles harder to get the extra oxygen, raising anxiety levels even further –another negative feedback cycle.

The stress and tension associated with an asthma attack may freeze the movement of the lung diaphragm. This is a sheet of muscle that separates the thoracic and abdominal cavities. When it moves downwards, it creates a vacuum effect in the thoracic cavity that causes air to move into the lungs. This muscle is the most powerful of the breathing muscles. Once out of action, you have to rely on the intercoastal muscles in the thoracic cavity. These operate to get air in but only to the upper part of the lungs. If you are relying on intercoastal muscles, your breath will be shallow and fast.

One of the important things in an asthma attack is to keep the breathing as deep and relaxed as possible. This is much easier said than done because such breathing relies on the mind being calmed and focused, and the mind is often anything but calm during the period of an attack. Practising body–mind exercises like Tai Chi can provide assistance. The mind is like the body – the more you train it in a task, the easier that task is to do. If you have a regular exercise regime that involves you putting yourself in a relaxed state and keeping yourself there, then when you do have an asthma attack it is much easier to remain calm. The techniques are not difficult. They can be as simple as mentally watching and observing your breath as it flows into and out of the lungs.

There are two other things that you can do to make sure that your breathing remains as calm and relaxed as possible:

1. Make sure during an attack that the functioning of the lung diaphragm is not inhibited by your posture or by constrictive clothing and belts. Loosen any tight clothing. The back should be straight. A curved spine will compress the thoracic cavity. Lying down is not a good idea. When standing or sitting in an upright position, the internal organs are pulled downwards by gravity and it is much easier for the lung diaphragm to move downwards into the abdominal cavity. When you are lying down, the internal organs roll back against the lung diaphragm and it has to work harder. If you must lie down, try to do so on a tilted surface so that the head is higher than the feet. Note that it is the slope of the body torso that is important – raising the head on a pillow or dropping the feet over the side of the bed is not going to help. Rather, place a pillow under the shoulders (but make sure the head is properly supported).
2. To assist in expelling air (which can be a problem in asthmatic attacks), it can help to place the palms on the upper abdomen under the rib cage (fingers pointing towards each other and almost touching), and press gently inwards and upwards with each exhalation.

One of the best things to do is make sure that the lung diaphragm is functioning properly prior to any attacks. You can establish this by performing the tests outlined in Part 4 of this book. Breathing using the lung diaphragm is often referred to as abdominal or diaphragmatic breathing and the techniques for this are one of the first things taught in Tai Chi.

REDUCTION IN THE NEGATIVE SECONDARY CONSEQUENCES OF ASTHMA

The negative consequences that can flow from asthma include:

- increased stress levels;
- depression (the mood, not the medical condition);
- social isolation.

REDUCTION IN STRESS LEVELS

The way that Tai Chi acts to reduce stress levels has already been discussed at some length. See above exercises for control over stress levels that arise during the onset of an asthma attack. They are most important, as stress will magnify the severity of the attack. Obviously such things as nasal breathing may not be practical during an attack but keeping the breath deep and long rather than fast and short will help. Also important is to keep tension out of the shoulders and waist. The first is achieved with either shoulder rolls or conscious lowering of the shoulders. The second by keeping the back straight.

REDUCTION IN DEPRESSION AND LOW VITALITY

We have already looked at how posture, eye positioning, breathing and mental visualisation can offset a feeling of depression or tiredness. Since the feeling of well-being will certainly be threatened during or after an asthma attack, using these techniques at this time can be very helpful.

REDUCTION IN SOCIAL ISOLATION

Social isolation refers to the fact that people don't want to be alone – they want to belong. They do not want to be different to friends, peers and family. Unfortunately, asthma often seems to require behaviour that makes the sufferer feel separate and isolated. Being part of groups made up of asthmatics and other people with breathing difficulties may provide critical support to the individual, but those with asthma also need to belong to other non-asthmatic mainstream groups or they will fall into the trap of defining themselves in terms of their condition. When an asthmatic person joins a Tai Chi group, they are joining a group made up of general members of the community.

There is yet a further advantage to practising Tai Chi. While the positive impacts that the exercise can make on your asthma may be your initial objective, you are also learning a valuable life skill that will be of benefit to you in many ways. So you don't have to see Tai Chi as yet another reduction in the quality of life that asthma may cause. It is not just another medicine to be taken, or another drain on your resources and time. Rather, you will find that Tai Chi can be a fascinating and enjoyable experience, an art and talent that you can take and develop throughout your life. It will mix you with people of all ages and interests. It is one way to fight back against the social isolation that asthma can otherwise impose.

IMPROVEMENT IN THE DIGESTIVE PROCESS AND THE UPTAKE OF BENEFICIAL MICRONUTRIENTS

An interesting indirect benefit of lowering stress is related to the impact of stress on vitamin A levels. Vitamin A is necessary to a number of bodily processes including the manufacture of adrenalin. (Adrenalin is often used to assist the easing of an asthmatic attack.) When one is stressed, one tends to use more adrenalin and hence more vitamin A. If one's diet is only providing just enough vitamin A, then being continually stressed may result in a shortage of this vitamin. There are certainly reports that indicate that some sufferers of asthma have experienced dramatic reductions in the incidence of asthmatic attacks through taking large daily doses of vitamin A. However, if the deficiency could be remedied by relaxation techniques rather than increased doses of vitamin A, this would obviously be preferable.

Stress has a further impact on Vitamin A levels in that stress tends to interfere with digestion. This is again a consequence of a short-term/long-term health trade-off. Digestion is about future health, so when the body initiates the stress response, it channels resources (such as the blood used to absorb digestive products) away from the digestive system to other systems that can have more impact on immediate survival (such as the cardiovascular and muscular systems). The whole process of digestion and assimilation may slow. Even at low levels of stress, there is a significant degradation of digestive function and one of the more vulnerable processes seems to be that which involves the absorption of vitamin A. So the more we can control stress the better.

As well as the direct absorption of vitamin A, the body can also manufacture its own vitamin A if provided with foods rich in a substance known as carotene. Not surprisingly, the main source of carotene is carrots. Again stress seems to threaten this conversion process. Consuming a reasonable quantity of carrots or carrot juice and remaining unstressed may therefore offer another way to reduce the incidence of asthmatic attacks.

Note Large doses of vitamin A can cause other problems. (This matter is dealt with more fully in the Nutrition section of Part 4.)

The How and Why of the ABMM Program

The fundamental principles or techniques of the ABMM program exercises are:

- posture;
- 'silk-like' movement;
- body-mind integration;
- awareness;
- Tai Chi breathing.

You might be surprised not to see the word 'relaxation' mentioned here but that is really because the concept of relaxation is so fundamental that each of these techniques could just have easily have been written:

- relaxation through posture;
- relaxation through 'silk-like' movement;
- relaxation through body-mind integration;
- relaxation through awareness;
- relaxation through Tai Chi breathing.

Relaxation and stress can be considered as two sides of the same coin in that one side of the coin always faces up. You are either relaxed or you are stressed. Since, if you are an asthmatic, being stressed will worsen your condition, it is important that you understand what 'relaxation' really means as opposed to how you may have seen it portrayed on the TV and other media!

What is relaxation?

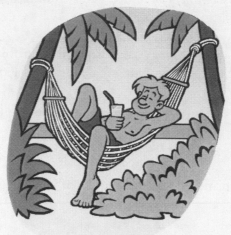

'STRESSFUL' RELAXATION

Relaxation is a term that causes all sorts of problems because different people mean quite different things when they speak of relaxation. To the ordinary person, the type of images that spring to mind when the subject of relaxation comes up are the images of lying on a beach, reclining in a hammock or some form of collapsed inactivity. The last image we tend to summon up when thinking of relaxation is the image of ourselves engaged in physical exercise. However, if you ever have the misfortune to be confined to bed for an extended period, you will soon find out exactly what that does to your body and how *stressed* it becomes from such 'relaxing activity'! One of the worst types of torture is to confine a person in a cramped position where they cannot stretch or move.

One important reason that hospitals try to get people up and about as soon as possible after hospitalisation or surgery is because it is healthier for us to be up and moving as soon as it is safe for us to do so. Prolonged inactivity leads to all sorts of complications. The muscular system degenerates, along with the ability to properly maintain blood pressure during the mildest activity. The immune system suffers as the movement of lymph fluid (which depends on body movement) slows. Even breathing is more difficult, as in the prone position the weight of the abdominal organs presses against the lung diaphragm. However, one should be careful not to leap to the contrary improper view that we should avoid lying down as much as possible. The fact is that stress is reduced and we are in our most relaxed state when there is a proper balance between activity and rest. Hence true relaxation is the continual search for a balance in activities and lifestyle that delivers optimum health.

Therefore if we re-look at the 'stressful relaxation' diagram above, we now see:

- faster, shallower breathing due to compression of lungs (increasing chance of asthma attack and raising anxiety levels);
- weakened cardiovascular system due to deterioration of muscles;
- increased pressure on heart because of inactivity in venous blood return system;
- under-performing immune system;
- decalcification of skeletal system (perhaps leading to osteoporosis) because of lack of weight-bearing exercise;
- increased risk of depression. (Depression is statistically greater in those less active.)

Perhaps the picture does not look quite as attractive as it once did!

To avoid confusion about what relaxation is, I have taken to using the term 'dynamic relaxation' to describe the type of relaxation being sought in this program, as opposed to the 'passive relaxation' that is involved with inactivity.

The ABMM program exercises recognise that the human body and mind are built around two basic response systems – the 'relaxation response' and the 'stress response' (sometimes called the flight or fight response). To better understand what these responses are designed to achieve, it is perhaps better to think of them as the 'long-term survival response' and the 'short-term survival response'.

THE 'RELAXATION' OR 'LONG-TERM SURVIVAL' RESPONSE

Here the body's energies and resources are focused towards keeping the body healthy as long as possible. This is the 'healing' mode, the state where the body's energies and resources are directed inward for repair, maintenance and growth. The energies of the body go to such things as the immune system, which defends us against disease and infection, and the digestive system, which nurtures and maintains us. It is the state where our organs and metabolic systems operate in a balanced and harmonious fashion that minimises long-term damage and strain on organs and tissues.

Tai Chi-based exercises are one of the few exercise systems that are designed to operate with the body remaining in the 'relaxation response'. Most other exercise systems, particularly those where the focus is on either competing against other people or various standards (composed of time, distance, height, etc), move the body into the stress response.

THE 'STRESS' OR 'SHORT-TERM SURVIVAL' RESPONSE

The stress response was evolved to deal with life-threatening situations, even if this required operating in a mode that shortened one's total life expectancy. This is a reasonable trade-off. If a large bull is charging towards you then it makes sense that your body becomes much more concerned about surviving the next few seconds than it is about surviving the next few decades.

In the stress response, the body's resources are withdrawn from systems such as the immune and digestive systems and redirected outward to muscular and energy-producing systems. Organs and metabolic processes are geared up to a level that ensures the body's short-term peak performance, no matter what the long-term damage done to organ and body systems. Blood is thickened and withdrawn from surface tissues and organs not essential to short-term survival so that not too much of this vital fluid is lost in the case of injury.

The stress response is like slamming on the brakes or flooring the accelerator when driving a car. It may get you out of an emergency situation, but it dramatically increases the risk of mechanical failure and accident if used as a standard driving technique. Unfortunately our bodies have not yet evolved to deal with today's modern environment and lifestyle. These continually create stimuli that put the body into stress response even though the situations are not life-threatening. In fact, the body's response to modern stresses is usually counterproductive.

Just think, when did getting stressed help in an exam or interview situation? Did being stressed improve how you handled that long traffic jam, the car breakdown, the ATM eating your credit card? So it's a lose-lose situation. Not only is there no real benefit to be gained and balanced off against the long-term damage that is being done, but the stress response usually makes things worse.

Does this mean that I am totally opposed to ever being stressed? Should we not compete in sports and business? Is having to meet a target or deadline bad for us? Not at all. The stress we feel when we abseil down a cliff, take a parachute jump or stand up in front of that audience to deliver a speech can provide an edge and focus that allows us to achieve more than we otherwise could. It can be stimulating and exhilarating. There are also often-significant benefits derived from such exercises through the improvement of cardiovascular and other body functions. The danger is when such exercises simply serve as an aggravation of an already overstressed life and lead to the worsening of existing problems. The trick is to use the response correctly and to be able to relax quickly.

For instance, if you are a rugby league player running towards the try line with half the other team thundering behind you, the stress response can be a real advantage that gives you an edge. But being in the stress response as you see a ball arcing towards you that you desperately want to catch can virtually guarantee a fumble as your hand and arms stiffen! There is a lot of emphasis in this book on the relaxation response as opposed to the stress response but that is because firstly, it is a trigger and aggravator of asthma attacks and secondly, while we are all pretty good at generating stress, most of us have a lot to learn about generating relaxation.

If as a person with asthma you do participate in a physically exertive (stressful) sport, then the practice of ABMM-based exercises can provide you with techniques that will be useful and that, if used in sensible combination with other sporting activities, can avoid or offset some of these activities' negative effects. At the same time, practice of these exercises can actually improve your sporting performance and reduce the risk of an exercise-triggered asthma attack.

Further benefits from learning exercise relaxation techniques

The techniques that achieve the relaxation response from exercise can be applied to most activities in life such as work, school and recreation.

One of the great things about the ABMM exercises is that once their practice becomes a part of your regular routine, the techniques start to become second-nature. They become sub-consciously applied in many other areas of life, helping to ensure that your body and mind remain as relaxed as possible throughout your day – not just during the time when you practise the exercises.

There is a further stress-related benefit to be derived from Tai Chi relaxation techniques. This arises from the fact that the nature of the stimuli that causes stress responses in today's lifestyle and environment generally does not result in the release of stress. For example, we can guess that our average caveman became somewhat stressed when he found a sabre-toothed tiger close behind him. The flight or fight that subsequently erupted would, if the caveman survived, release any muscular tension built up and metabolise any adrenalin and other stress hormones that had been produced. Today, however, when we are caught in a traffic jam or queue, frustrated by the non-appearance of a meal we ordered, or suffering unfair criticism from our boss, there is no opportunity to release the built-up stress. This means that not only do we suffer stress during the situation but for a long time after as well. These stored tensions have a number of deleterious effects, including a tendency to become more stressed (a negative feedback cycle). ABMM program exercises break this cycle by teaching us how to release these stored tensions.

The removal of stored muscular tension has particular benefit for asthmatics as two key areas where the body stores stress are in the shoulders and the abdominal areas. Tension in these areas can constrict and interfere with breathing, reducing the available lung capacity. Not only is the increase in available lung capacity a positive benefit in asthmatic attacks but the slower breathing cycle that results from utilisation of this extra lung capacity can in itself reduce the level of stress and anxiety that is present (thus initiating a positive rather than negative feedback cycle).

POSTURE
We tend to think of posture as simply keeping a straight back to look better. However, posture has an intimate relationship with not only how we look but also how we think and feel; how balanced we are

physically, mentally and emotionally. Furthermore, posture affects our breathing, digestion and our circulation of blood and lymph fluid. It is intimately tied up with our whole sense. It is of crucial importance to those with asthma.

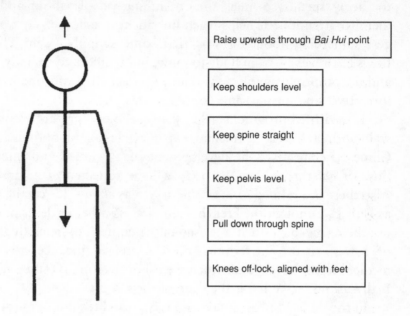

Raise upwards through *Bai Hui* point

Keep shoulders level

Keep spine straight

Keep pelvis level

Pull down through spine

Knees off-lock, aligned with feet

A 'posture' experiment

Posture affects mood dramatically. If you find this difficult to believe then try the following experiment:

- Stand with your feet shoulder-width apart. Tilt your head forward, draw your shoulders slightly inwards and fix your eyes firmly on a spot on the floor between your feet.
- Now, without straightening up or raising your eyes, speak enthusiastically to a friend or family member about a recent enjoyable experience such as a holiday, a meal, or a meeting with an old friend. Try to recapture your mood and feeling and convey how much you enjoyed the experience. (If you can't think of an enjoyable experience then you definitely need Tai Chi!) How do you feel?
- Now straighten the spine, feeling as though your head is supported by a string connected to the crown of your head. Relax the whole

body down from this point, look ahead, and deliver the same speech. Notice the difference in how you feel.

Posture affects the way you think and behave. Why else do you think the army spends so much time marching people about and standing them to attention? It helps teach uncritical obedience. That might suggest something about the way that some schools teach! The process flows both ways – from body to mind and from mind to body. Rigorous and uncompromising persons tend to reflect their attitude in their posture. Two sides of the same coin.

The ABMM program teaches you a relaxed upright posture that sits well with a feeling of mental expansiveness and optimism. From a Chinese perspective, the development of a relaxed and unconstricted flow of *chi* throughout the body will be reflected in mental attitude. Also there is a refined form of *chi* known as *shen*. This can be translated as 'spirit', although the French 'élan vital' is a better description. If you use the term 'spirit' then it is used in the context of being 'high-spirited' or 'low-spirited'. The term has no religious significance, it is a Chinese medical term. In the West when we ask a person how they feel, we are really asking is, 'What is the state of their *shen*?'

In the ABMM program we use recognised techniques for raising the *shen* and when it is raised, the mood of depression disappears and an optimistic outgoing mood is encouraged. These techniques are borrowed from Tai Chi and are another reason why Tai Chi is regarded as an 'internal art'.

SILK-LIKE MOVEMENT
In a similar manner to posture, the nature of our movement is intimately related to our degree of relaxation and all the benefits that are attached to the relaxation response. The Chinese have long referred to a type of movement they call *mian* or 'silk-like' movement. The name is derived both from the soft, flowing nature of silk and the way that the silken thread used to be drawn manually from the silkworm's cocoon. Any jerkiness, any sudden changes in speed or direction, and the delicate silk thread was broken. Your relaxation is as delicate as the silk thread. Move suddenly, move jerkily and it will be broken as you move into the stress response.

One useful piece of imagery for creating silk-like movement is to imagine that when moving your hands some very rare butterflies have landed on each of your hands, and you do not want to disturb them before you can show somebody.

Transitions, from upward to downward, from left to right, from stillness to movement, from movement to stillness, are the areas to focus on, as this is where jerkiness and a break in the thread of your relaxation is likely to occur.

BODY–MIND INTEGRATION

Body–mind integration is about making sure that the body and mind are doing the same thing. While this may sound simple, one of the greatest problems in exercising is being 'distracted'. Two methods of achieving this focus are to either keep your mind on breathing patterns or on the movement of *chi*.

'Where the mind goes the *chi* flows', goes the old Chinese expression and modern research would also support the fact that when we are 'in touch' with our bodies we can achieve quite spectacular results. But if we are putting our mind in touch with our bodies, we want to be sure that the mind is saying the right things! An important part of body–mind integration is positive thinking. When you perform your exercises, maintain positive visualisation. Focus on how good you feel and how much better you are getting rather than 'avoiding the next asthma attack'.

AWARENESS

This may sound like a contradiction to body-mind integration because it requires external awareness. But there is a world of difference between doing a movement while you are thinking of what you are going to say to your boss to get a pay rise and doing a movement while being aware of the sights and sounds that surround you. The fact is that your sensory organs are part of your body and need to be involved in the exercise that you are performing.

You might find that the process of 'shutting out' is actually a stressful one. Not only do we generally express our feeling of relaxing by doing such things as listening to music, tasting good food, smelling the flowers and looking at the countryside but doing these things will also tend to bring about relaxation.

This is just one reason why we should look closely not only at the environment that we exercise in but any environment in which we spend significant proportions of our time.

TAI CHI BREATHING

This is the name given to diaphragmatic breathing where the breathing is not forced but responsive, and the air is breathed into and out of the nose. The two most beneficial techniques in this program are the breathing techniques and the stress management or relaxation techniques. As can be seen from the following analysis, breathing and relaxation are linked in an either mutually reinforcing or mutually destructive manner.

The prime objective of the breathing process is to maintain appropriate levels of oxygen and carbon dioxide within the blood. As metabolic activity increases (through exercise for instance), oxygen is drawn out of the blood at a faster rate and the lungs must breathe in more air to replenish the oxygen, which has been concerted converted into the metabolic waste product of carbon dioxide.

It all sounds pretty simple, but in fact the breathing or respiration process is amazingly subtle and sophisticated. Breathing is important not only to our continued existence but also to our quality of life and state of vitality, so much so that it warrants our full understanding.

Getting Rid of Some Misconceptions

Perhaps the major misconception to get rid of is that if we need oxygen to live then the more oxygen we get the better. This is incorrect — too much oxygen in the blood is as bad as too little. Oxygen at higher levels than the body is programmed to maintain is a poison that can seriously damage the body!

The next misconception to get rid of is that if carbon dioxide is a waste product then we had better get rid of as much of it as we can (usually by forced exhalation). Lowering carbon dioxide levels in the blood too far results in hyperventilation and interferes with a number of metabolic processes.

The human body has developed sophisticated chemical sensors that measure the chemical constitution of the blood to ensure that the appropriate level of oxygen and carbon dioxide is maintained. We breathe faster as we exercise because these sensors measure the rising proportion of carbon dioxide in the blood and trigger the inhalation process more frequently.

We should no more attempt to consciously interfere with the volume of air that these sensors determine is required in a given period of time than we should try to consciously interfere with the amount of blood that our heart is pumping. Unfortunately, it is much easier to consciously interfere with our breath than our heart rate. However, while our conscious brain can override the automatic breathing process, it has no way of determining what the oxygen needs of the body are, and will almost certainly cause us to breathe in either too much or too little.

What do we need breathing exercises for, if not for more oxygen or less carbon dioxide?

On the face of it, it might sound as though we should not be doing breathing exercises at all, but the trick lies in understanding how to consciously influence the breathing pattern without changing the volume of air that the chemical sensors have determined is appropriate to breathe in over a given period of time. There are still ways that we can influence the process because the volume of air we breathe in during a given time depends on two factors:

- the volume of air we inhale with each in-breath;
- the number of breaths we take in each minute.

The existence of these two factors allows us to use our conscious mind and our automatic breathing process together. If we, for instance, consciously slow our breathing, the automatic breathing system responds by deepening the breath to make sure that the total volume of air breathed in over a given period of time remains at the appropriate level. On the other hand, if we deepen our breathing, then our automatic breathing system reduces the number of breaths we take per minute so that, again, the total volume of air inhaled remains constant.

This means that we can focus on either deepening our breath or slowing our breath as long as we do not try to do both at the same time. Does it make any difference to the body whether we take 12 breaths of one amount of air per minute or six breaths of twice that amount? The answer is a very definite 'yes' because the breathing function does not operate in isolation to other body systems.

Most of us know that when we are anxious, nervous or afraid, we tend to breathe quickly and shallowly. This is an evolutionary device that shifts us into the stress response to prepare us for action. This made sense in those days when we lived in the forests and jungles; if we were consciously concerned or worried about something in the environment, then the body also had to be prepared for 'fight or flight'. This is what the stress response is designed to prepare us for. The stress response, however, has a large number of negative impacts on long-term health.

These negatives include such things as:

- shortening one's life because of increased wear and tear on body systems;
- increased risk of disease and infection because of the running down of the immune system;
- for asthmatics, increased chance of asthma attack and likelihood of increased severity of an asthma attack.

Of course, these negatives don't matter too much if the alternative is failing to survive the next few minutes! But why breathe in a manner that causes these problems if there is no survival benefit?

On the other hand, most of us know that when we are relaxed and at ease, our breathing tends to be slow and deep. This was another evolutionary response. If the conscious mind was relaxed and at ease then there was probably no imminent threat and the body could concern itself with growth and maintenance. Of course society has evolved faster than the body and even now most of the threats we face in a modern world are better handled in a relaxed rather than stressed state. Think driving, work relations, exams, etc. Do you perform these tasks better when you are stressed or relaxed?

So in Tai Chi breathing we seek either to consciously slow our breath or consciously deepen our breath but never both!

TECHNIQUES FOR CONSCIOUSLY SLOWING THE BREATH

Tai Chi has three very simple techniques for consciously slowing the breath:

- increasing the effective vital capacity of the lungs;
- breathing in and out through the nose;
- mental awareness of the breath.

When we correct our posture and release tensions from the muscles, the effective vital capacity of our lungs increases because the lungs are not being compressed by postural and muscular distortion.

When we breathe in and out through the nose, the nose simply cannot pass large volumes of air quickly so our breathing becomes slowed.

The simple act of becoming aware of the breath flowing into and out of the body slows down our breath rate. We are not consciously forcing the breath to be slower, we are simply becoming aware of the flow of air and how it feels as it passes through the nose, throat and lungs. We may become aware of the movements in the body torso, the rise and fall of the shoulders, the expansion and contraction of the abdomen, the wave-like motion that goes through the spine. Again, if we consciously try to create these, we only cause problems. It is the sense of listening with the senses that helps the breathing slow. As an example, just feel the difference in the texture of the different items of clothing that you are wearing at the moment.

I would suspect that while practising this awareness exercise, you found that your breathing was slowing. This is not because you consciously tried to slow the movement, but because you needed time to collect and evaluate the sensory data and your breathing automatically slowed to allow this to happen. The same process takes place in any breathing visualisation.

TECHNIQUES FOR CONSCIOUSLY DEEPENING THE BREATH

The deepness of the breath, that is the volume of air taken into the lungs at each breath, can be adversely affected by a number of factors:

- Tension in the shoulders (this reduces the amount by which the

upper lungs can be expanded).
- Curvature of the spine (which compresses internal organs and lungs together).
- Abdominal tension (which reduces the movement of the lung diaphragm; thus reducing the amount by which the lower lungs can be expanded).
- Stress or inactivity of the lung diaphragm (which again reduces lower lung capacity).

All of the above factors cause reduction in the effective capacity of the lungs. This means that more breaths must be taken per minute to maintain required oxygen levels in the blood, and, also of the faster breathing puts us back deeper into the stress response, establishing a negative feedback cycle that can be difficult to break.

There is another adverse impact of reduced lung capacity that should not be overlooked. The expansion and contraction of the lungs within the body torso creates an internal massaging effect that assists in:

- returning venous blood (depleted in oxygen and full of wastes and toxins) to the general circulatory system. This occurs when the lung diaphragm presses down on the internal organs, effectively squeezing out the venous blood;
- supplying arterial blood (full of oxygen and nutrients) to the internal organs. This occurs when the lung diaphragm moves upwards, reducing the pressure in the abdominal cavity and causing internal organs to expand by drawing in fresh blood;
- moving food through the intestinal tract, improving the digestive system;
- moving lymph fluid around the torso. Lymph fluid is important in maintaining an effective immune system.

Guidelines for Breathing Exercises

For the reasons explained earlier in Part 2, it is important that we do not force our breathing or over-breathe. If you follow the instructions to the exercises, this should not occur. However, if you find yourself becoming giddy or nauseous during breathing exercises, this is a symptom that your body's requirement for oxygen and your breathing are out of sync. If this occurs, sit quietly and let your body re-establish its' normal breathing rate. If the problem recurs each time you do breathing exercises, seek advice from your medical practitioner.

Do not try to fill your lungs more than about 70 to 80 per cent. You will know that you are doing this because there will be a feeling of distension in the chest and the air will tend to rush out when you start to breathe out — rather than flowing out gently or your chest will feel over-inflated and stressed. Also do not try to empty more air out of the lungs than is comfortable. Your chest should feel comfortable throughout the breathing cycle. This is a Tai Chi approach so your breath should be relaxed.

You will find that if you empty and fill your lungs too much, the change from in-breath to out-breath and vice versa will seem jerky and abrupt when it should be smooth and relaxed. The operative words in Tai Chi breathing are soft, quiet, smooth, relaxed and flowing.

BREATHING THROUGH THE NOSE
The benefits of breathing through the nose include:

- the encouragement of relaxation;
- protects lungs against infection;
- protects lungs against allergens;
- encouragement of the use of the lung diaphragm.

There are of course lots of other advantages to breathing through the nose that are of particular benefit to asthmatics. These are dealt with later in this book

PART 3

The Body–Mind
Exercise Session

Before you start the program let your doctor know!

Questions you need answered to carry out a successful body–mind exercise session

1. HOW IS A BODY–MIND EXERCISE SESSION STRUCTURED AND WHY?

The 'model' body-mind exercise session is structured as follows:

Exercise Number	Name of Exercise	Suggested Time for Exercise
Exercise 1	Quiet Standing/Sitting	2 minutes
Exercise 2	Shoulder Relaxation Exercises	3 minutes
Exercise 3	Swinging Arms	2 minutes
Exercise 4	Breathing Visualisations	4 minutes
Exercise 5	Abdominal Massage(s)	4 minutes
Exercise 6	Supplementary Optional Exercises	7 minutes
Exercise 7	Lung Meridan Acupressure Massage	3 minutes
Exercise 8	Opening the Chest	3 minutes
Exercise 9	Quiet Standing/Sitting	2 minutes
	Total	30 minutes

The objectives of each element are as follows:

1. QUIET STANDING/SITTING
Objective: Lowers stress levels, calms the mind, slows the breathing and heart rate, drops anxiety levels and corrects posture.

2. SHOULDER RELAXATION EXERCISES
Objective: Releases the tension stored in the shoulder area. Such tension causes postural distortions that interfere with breathing and raise anxiety levels. This type of tension needs to be removed prior to working on breathing and breathing visualisation.

3. SWINGING ARMS

Objective: Loosens up tensions in the waist area and allows the lung diaphragm to function properly. Swinging arms will also further loosen up tension in the shoulder area.

4. BREATHING VISUALISATIONS

Objective: Further slows the breathing while deepening the relaxation response, encouraging *chi* flow and positive visualisation within the mind.

5. ABDOMINAL MASSAGE

Objective: Continues the release of stresses and tensions in the abdominal area, allowing the lung diaphragm to function properly.

6. SUPPLEMENTARY OPTIONAL EXERCISES

Objective: Use of one or more optional exercises designed to strengthen the body and mind, particularly the immune and respiratory functions.

7. LUNG MERIDIAN ACUPRESSURE MASSAGE

Objective: To use the body's own energy to enhance the lung function.

8. OPENING THE CHEST EXERCISE

Objective: Generates a calm flow of energy through the body that can then be used in the Lung Acupressure techniques.

9. QUIET STANDING/SITTING

Objective: To ensure that after the focus on the lung points, we return to our daily activities with proper posture, breathing and mental focus.

2. CAN YOU VARY THE MAKE-UP OF THE BODY-MIND EXERCISE SESSION?

This is a 'model' that you can vary but it does have a very specific structure so it is best to carry out the body-mind exercise session in the order presented with all of the elements present. Even though the session is not strenuous, it has 'warm up' and 'cool down' elements to its structure.

To add variation, you can increase the time you spend on any element or even incorporate extra exercises from outside the program. Any exercise from the Tai Chi form – or *Ba Dua Gin, Shibashi Tai Chi Chi*

Kung, *Lotus* and *Tao Yin* – could be added to the program with benefit, provided they supplement rather than supplant the recommended exercises. Possibly you may even become fired up to learn a Tai Chi form. (A 'form' is simply an interconnected sequence of movements that adhere to Tai Chi principles. The most common forms are the *Yang*, *Chen* and *Wu* forms.) This is probably the time you might consider becoming involved with one of the AATC's regular courses. If this is not practicable, you might like to give us a call and we will discuss some possible variations that you might make to the program. The Appendices also provide a resource list that may be of use in this regard.

The advantages of participating in a class, apart from the fun of performing in a group, include access to a qualified instructor who is constantly evaluating your progress. Let your instructor know that you are undertaking the program and the instructor will be able to make suggestions that speed up your progress and improve the benefits that you obtain. If you are too shy to do this, the ABMM program itself helps you identify those movements and techniques in classes that are going to be of most use to you from an asthma perspective.

3. HOW LONG SHOULD EACH BODY–MIND EXERCISE SESSION BE?

The body–mind exercise session should extend for at least 30 minutes and should be uninterrupted.

The initiation of the relaxation response and its maintenance for a period of at least 20 minutes is most important. Mentally we can relax quite quickly. We judge the state of mental relaxation by the types of brainwaves that are produced, with alpha waves indicating a profound level of relaxation. It has been shown that after a little practice most people can produce alpha waves after a few seconds of proper mental focus. The body, however, is basically biochemical in nature and it takes time for the levels of stressor chemicals such as adrenalin to be reduced, but generally this can be achieved if the mind remains relaxed for 20 minutes. If both the body and the mind are relaxed at the end of the session then the period of time before we become stressed again will be extended. This is not just a matter of feeling good longer; health is dependent on the ratio of time that we spend in the relaxation response compared to the stress response. The higher this ratio the better.

Studies have shown that when you take a group of people who have just performed a period of relaxing exercise and give them a stressful task to perform, the exercise that shows the slowest increase in stress levels is Tai Chi.

4. HOW MANY BODY–MIND EXERCISE SESSIONS SHOULD I DO EACH WEEK?

It is suggested that, in the early stages, at least three body–mind exercise sessions per week are necessary to see any real improvement. But do not go to the other extreme. Most of us get very enthusiastic about things when we first start off but more exercise does not necessarily mean you will obtain more benefits. An old Tai Chi story explains the fallacy:

A keen student once approached his Tai Chi master to ask how long it would be before he would succeed in mastering his Tai Chi. The Master asked to watch his Tai Chi and questioned him about his training program. After some deliberation the Master then advised the student that it would take him about two years more to master the Tai Chi form. The student was clearly disappointed about the length of time and asked the Master how long it would take if he doubled the training he was doing. The Master replied that was a much more difficult question but that he would think about three years. The student was aghast and asked how long it would take if he spent every possible moment that he could in training his Tai Chi. 'Ah,' said the Master, 'that is the easiest question yet – with that approach you would never master the art of Tai Chi!'

The point is that so many of the benefits of the ABMM program flow from getting the body into a relaxed state. This is the first objective – the more you take a relaxed approach to the ABMM program, the better it will work. But remember relaxation means 'Dynamic Relaxation' and that means you still have to do things – just make sure that you do them in a relaxed manner!

5. WHAT IS THE BEST TIME OF THE DAY TO DO A BODY-MIND EXERCISE SESSION?

The body-mind exercise session can be run just as effectively in the morning, afternoon or evening. Try not to do the session just after you have eaten. Leave about 30 minutes or more, depending on the size of the meal. Also, do not force yourself to exercise in periods when you are hungry or stressed.

The most important thing you can do to assure the success of your ABMM program is to schedule a fixed time slot for the body-mind exercise session. Experience has shown that if you do the session 'when you have time', somehow you will find that time never materialises and the ABMM program fails before it ever really gets going.

Getting a group together to practise would be very beneficial as it helps ensure that you will make the time because you will not want to let other members of the group down. Somehow that is always more important than letting ourselves down!

6. WHERE IS THE BEST PLACE TO DO A BODY-MIND EXERCISE SESSION?

You can perform the body-mind exercise session indoors or out. The best place is one where you can exercise undisturbed and the air is fresh. The more pleasant the location, the better you will feel after exercising and the greater the benefits you will get. Here are some 'helpful hints':

- You don't need much room to carry out the exercise program. If you are exercising indoors then it can be carried out in most lounge rooms if you have about two square metres per person of clear space. Alternatively you could easily find the space on a verandah or in a garden.
- Make sure that whatever place you choose is free from draughts or exposure to damp and extreme heat, cold or wind.
- Turn off the mobile phone and take the phone off the hook. Make it clear to family and friends that they are welcome to join in, but that this is your time for your health.

7. SHOULD YOU USE MUSIC IN A BODY-MIND EXERCISE SESSION?

You may find it advantageous to play some relaxing music (but avoid anything with a regular beat – such music actually stimulates). If you like to perform your exercise to the sound of the sea, the breeze in the trees or the sound of water in a fountain or stream, that is fine too. Remember that these days you do not need a beach or forest on your doorstep because there are many tapes and CDs of relaxing natural sounds available.

One advantage of playing relaxing music as you exercise is that the subconscious quickly grows to associate the pleasant feelings of relaxation experienced during the exercise session with the music. This means that when you play the music at other times, your body will tend to relax, even if you are not performing the body-mind exercise session. But don't be surprised if you get the urge to get up and exercise!

Actually, you can use this to your own advantage for those exercise days when you really don't feel like going through the session. (Yes, it does happen to us all!) Just turn on the music a few minutes before the time of your exercise session and you may suddenly feel yourself 'in the mood' for exercise.

8. WHAT CLOTHING SHOULD YOU WEAR IN A BODY–MIND EXERCISE SESSION?

As long as clothing is loose and comfortable, it will suffice. Shoes should be flat-soled.

9. HOW DO YOU KNOW WHETHER TO USE THE SITTING OR STANDING VERSIONS OF THE BODY–MIND EXERCISES?

The standing versions of the exercise will definitely have better health benefits if you can stand comfortably for 30 minutes. If this is not possible then the next best thing is the sitting version provided.

If you use the sitting version, be careful with your choice of chair. This should comply with the following requirements:

- it should be firm and stable;
- it should allow free movement of the body and arms;
- the seat should be flat – not tilted back towards a back support;
- when you sit on the chair, your heels and toes should rest comfortably on the ground with your upper leg parallel to the ground.

10. ARE THERE ANY OTHER THINGS THAT CAN BE DONE TO IMPROVE THE BENEFITS OF THE BODY-MIND EXERCISE SESSION?

Access to a mirror where you can check your posture can be of assistance when you do not have an instructor to call your attention to postural defects.

A relaxing aroma such as lavender can help you to relax during exercise sessions.

Exercise 1   Opening: Quiet Standing/Sitting

Refer to previous page for details on whether the Quiet Sitting or Standing version should be used.

PHYSICAL MOVEMENT — QUIET STANDING

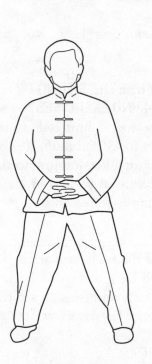
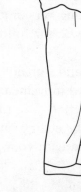

Front View   **Side View**

To establish the Quiet Standing position, go through the steps listed below in the order that they appear. You should make sure that if you are wearing shoes, they are loose and comfortable with flat soles, like sandshoes or joggers. High-heeled shoes introduce postural distortion that can have particularly bad effects for people with asthma.

- Place your feet shoulder-width apart. The feet should be parallel with the toes pointing to the front.

  Throughout the Quiet Standing, try to feel as though the weight is equally distributed between both feet and centred between the toes and heels. If the weight comes forward on the toes, backward onto the heels or sideways onto one foot or the other, it will cause muscular tension and postural distortion. Check that your toes just rest gently on the ground and are not clenched or upturned.

- Imagine that there is a string attached to the crown of your head and that your whole body can hang down from this point with the weight of your body supported by the string.

  While this step is included primarily to ensure correct physical posture, it is also important from an energy viewpoint. The point where our 'imaginary' string attaches is the 'Bai Hui' acupoint. When we focus our attention on this point we raise the body's energy and gain a heightened sense of vitality. In Chinese terms we are 'raising the shen'. This is particularly important for those with asthma since it helps to counter depression and unblock emotions. This effect can be enhanced by feeling that one is 'smiling' through the eyes.

- Now allow yourself to be 'lowered' by the imaginary string until the knees bend naturally into the 'off-lock' position.

If this seems difficult, experiment by imagining yourself being alternately raised and lowered by the imaginary string and see how, as you imagine yourself drawn up, the knees seem to straighten without you consciously putting tension into the legs. As you imagine yourself lowered, your knees will automatically bend and you sink only far enough for the knees to come forward about two or three centimetres.

- Make sure the pelvis is relaxed.

  Many people tilt the pelvis backward. This causes a pronounced curve in the lumbar area that causes many postural distortions and can lead to back problems. This is particularly important for those with asthma because the postural distortions impact on the ability to perform proper diaphragmatic breathing. Also, with the tensions and stresses associated with asthma, those with this condition are more likely to have this postural problem in the first place.

  If you are not sure whether your pelvis is correctly positioned, place your palms over the curve of your pelvic bones, thumbs forward, then tilt your pelvis forward. If you rub the back of one hand down over the lower spine, it should now seem flatter. With the pelvis in the right position, the stomach will tend to feel 'folded'. Despite this sensation you will find that it is much easier to use diaphragmatic breathing than when the pelvis is tucked back.

- First relax the arms by allowing them to hang loosely by the sides, then gently lift the shoulders three or four centimetres before allowing them to sink down into a 'comfortable position'. As you complete this, stretch the fingertips slowly downwards towards the floor. Then, keeping the fingers extended, bring the hands inwards over the abdomen so that the right palm rests on the surface of the abdomen just below the navel and the left palm is placed over the back of the right palm.

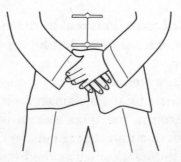

Make sure that the elbow joints are relaxed. Placing the hand in this position is important in encouraging the flow of energy. The hands are actually over an acupoint called chi hai, *which is associated with the extraction of energy from the breathing process. In this position, you will also be able to focus on the gentle expansion and contraction of the abdomen that occurs with each inhalation and exhalation when the lung diaphragm is functioning correctly.*

- The mouth should be closed but more through bringing the lips together rather than the teeth. Bringing the teeth together brings tension into the lower jaw. The tip of the tongue can rest against the back of the upper set of teeth or on the hard palate if this is comfortable.

Placing the mouth in this position achieves a number of things. First it ensures that one is breathing through the nose, not the mouth. The importance of this has already been discussed at length. The position of the tongue creates a better connection between the du mo *and* ren mai *meridians, the major energy circuit of the body. It also causes increased salivation, which improves both digestion and protection against infection.*

- Relax the face particularly around the eyes (you can do this by slightly tensing the facial muscles then releasing the tension away).

PHYSICAL MOVEMENT – QUIET SITTING

To achieve the Quiet Sitting position, go through the steps listed below in the order that they appear. You should make sure that if you are wearing shoes, they are loose and comfortable with flat soles like sand-shoes or joggers. High-heeled shoes introduce postural distortions, even in sitting positions, which can have particularly bad effects for people with asthma. (See answer to question 9 for requirements for chair.)

- Sit on the front third of the chair or stool so that your thighs are parallel with the ground, with your feet shoulder-width apart, supporting perhaps one-third of the body weight. The feet should be parallel, with the toes pointing to the front.

Throughout the Quiet Sitting, try to feel as though the weight on the feet is equally distributed between both feet and centred between the toes and heels of each foot. If the weight comes forward on the toes, backward onto the heels or sideways onto one foot or the other it will cause muscular tension and postural distortion. Check that your toes just rest gently on the ground and are not clenched or upturned. The remainder of your weight is supported by the but-tocks. Do not lean backwards.

- Imagine that there is a string attached to the crown of your head and that your whole body can hang down from this point with the weight of your body supported by the string.

While this step is primarily included to ensure correct physical pos-ture, it is also important from an energy viewpoint. The point where our 'imaginary' string attaches is the 'bai hui' acupoint. When we focus our attention on this point we raise the body's energy and gain a heightened sense of vitality. In Chinese terms we are 'raising the shen'. This is particularly important for those with asthma since it helps to counter depression and unblock emotions. This effect can be enhanced by feeling that one is 'smiling' through the eyes.

- Make sure the pelvis and lumbar area is relaxed.

When sitting down, many people either slump the pelvis and lumbar vertebra backwards or strain upwards through the back creating an exaggerated lumbar curve. This is particularly important for those with asthma because the postural distortions impact on the ability to perform proper diaphragmatic breathing. Also, with the tensions and stresses associated with asthma, those with this condition are more likely to have these postural problems in the first place.

If you're not sure whether your pelvis is correctly positioned, draw in the back slightly until you can rub the back of one hand down over the lower spine without feeling any curvature. Without adjusting the spine, relax the abdominal muscles. With the pelvis in the right position, the stomach will tend to feel 'folded'. Despite this sensation, you will find that it is much easier to use diaphragmatic breathing than when the lumbar area is straight without being tense.

- First relax the arms by allowing them to hang loosely by the sides then gently lift the shoulders three or four centimetres before allowing them to sink down into a 'comfortable position'. As you complete this, stretch the fingertips slowly downwards towards the floor. Then, keeping the fingers extended, bring the hands inwards over the abdomen so that the left palm rests on the surface of the abdomen just below the navel and the right palm is placed over the back of the left palm.

Make sure that the elbow joints are relaxed. Placing the hands in this position is important in encouraging the flow of energy. The hands are actually over an acupoint called chi hai, *which is associated with the extraction of energy from the breathing process. In this position, you will also be able to focus on the gentle expansion and contraction of the abdomen that occurs with each inhalation and exhalation when the lung diaphragm is functioning correctly.*

- The mouth should be closed, but more through bringing the lips together rather than the teeth. Bringing the teeth together brings tension into the lower jaw. The tip of the tongue can rest against the back of the upper set of teeth or on the hard palate if this is comfortable.

Placing the mouth in this position achieves a number of things. First it ensures that one is breathing through the nose not the mouth. The importance of this has already been discussed at length. The position of the tongue creates a better connection between the du mo and ren mai meridians, the major energy circuit of the body. It also causes increased salivation, which improves both digestion and protection against infection.

- Relax the face particularly around the eyes (you can do this by slightly tensing the facial muscles then releasing the tension away).

MENTAL IMAGERY AND BREATHING SYNCHRONISATION

If you have followed the above instructions, you will have become very aware of the position and posture of your body. This integration of mind and body is most important and you should attempt to maintain it while in the Quiet Standing/Sitting position.

When you are satisfied that your body is correctly positioned, allow your mind to become quiet and still. Errant thoughts will sometimes appear but do not let this concern you; just let those thoughts float away. It can sometimes help to count your breaths.

Remember, do not control your breaths. Just be aware of your body breathing and count each in-breath and out-breath as it happens. If you watch your breathing, you will find that it almost naturally slows, and as it slows you become more relaxed. Count off at least 15 full breaths before moving on to the second exercise.

GRANDMASTER KHOR'S KEY POINTS

1. Feel as though the body is lifted through the crown of the head and all the muscles and flesh of the body hang down.
2. Sink the *chi* by focusing on deep diaphragmatic breathing.
3. Tuck the tailbone under so that the spine has a gentle stretch.
4. Relax, relax, relax!

BENEFITS

The major benefits of the Quiet Standing/Sitting exercise are:

- the initiation of the relaxation response, the benefits of which were detailed earlier;
- the correction of posture with specific benefits for breathing;
- the adoption of Tai Chi-based breathing.

The reader might also consider that any opportunity for practising Quiet Standing/Sitting during the daily routine of life can only be of benefit. When you are standing in queues it is relatively easy to practice Quiet Standing without drawing attention to yourself. Simply leave the hands at the sides rather than placing them on the abdomen. You kill two birds with one stone – instead of having to be frustrated about waiting times, you can now use them to become even more relaxed.

Exercise 2 Shoulder Relaxation

CONTINUITY

Maintain the posture and breathing from quiet standing, relax the hands slowly to the side.

PHYSICAL MOVEMENT AND BREATHING SYNCHRONISATION

- Roll both shoulders upward and forward in slow, smooth, gentle circles that synchronise with the breath. The upward, forward part of the shoulder roll is done on the in-breath and the downward backward part on the out-breath.

  Complete eight forward double shoulder rolls.

- Now reverse the motion rolling both shoulders backward, in smooth, gentle circles that synchronise with the breath. The upward backward part of the roll is done on the in-breath, the downward forward part of the roll is done on the out-breath.

  Complete eight backward double shoulder rolls.

- Keeping the left shoulder still, reverse the motion, rolling the right shoulder forward in slow, smooth, gentle circles that synchronise with the breath. The upward forward part of the shoulder roll is done on the in-breath, the downward backward part of the roll on the out-breath.

  Complete four forward right shoulder rolls.

- Keeping the left shoulder still, reverse the motion, rolling the right shoulder backward in smooth gentle circles that synchronise with the breath. The upward, backward part of the roll is done on the in-breath, the downward forward part is done on the out-breath.

  Complete four backward right shoulder rolls.

71

- Keeping the right shoulder still, roll the left shoulder forward in slow, smooth, gentle circles that synchronise with the breath. The upward forward part of the shoulder roll is done on the in-breath, the downward backward part on the out-breath.

Complete four forward left shoulder rolls.

- Keeping the right shoulder still, reverse the motion, rolling the left shoulder backward in smooth, gentle circles that synchronise with the breath. The upward backward part of the roll is done on the in-breath, the downward forward part on the out-breath.

Complete four backward left shoulder rolls.

- Now, roll the shoulders forward alternately. That is, when one shoulder is up, the other shoulder is down. Again use slow, smooth, gentle circles that synchronise with the breath. The upward forward part of the right shoulder roll is done on the in-breath, the downward backward part on the out-breath.

Complete eight forward alternate shoulder rolls.

- Reverse the motion, rolling the shoulders backward alternately. That is, when one shoulder is up, the other shoulder is down. Again use smooth gentle circles that synchronise with the breath. The upward backward part of the right shoulder roll is done on the in-breath, the downward forward part on the out-breath.

Complete eight backward alternate shoulder rolls

- On the in-breath, gently raise both shoulders. On the out-breath, lower the shoulders as gently to their natural resting position. On the next in-breath, gently stretch the fingertips down towards the ground. On the out-breath, slowly release the stretch and allow the shoulders to relax.

Repeat this entire cycle three times.

SITTING OPTION

All the above shoulder exercises can be performed in exactly the same manner from the Quiet Sitting position. Ensure that the chair being used allows the arms to hang down loosely at the sides.

MENTAL IMAGERY

Throughout this exercise, keep your mind focused on how the shoulders feel. Can you sense the movement of the bones, muscles and tendons in the shoulder area as you perform the exercise? Try to visualise the shoulder area becoming warmer and more fluid. Feel the circular motion being slow smooth and even. Using the mind in this way is one of the most important parts of this exercise – do not let your mind wander to other things!

GRANDMASTER KHOR'S KEY POINTS

1. Make sure that the arms remain relaxed at all times. There can be a tendency to use the elbows to push up the shoulder. This puts tension into the shoulder area rather than removing it. Rather, feel the shoulders lifting and lowering the arms.

2. Only roll the shoulders in a vertical plane. That is, the shoulders should not be brought inwards towards the neck as this, again, increases tension rather than removing it. The trick is to consciously focus on keeping your shoulders as far from your neck as you can without straining.

BENEFITS

These exercises release muscular tension stored in the shoulders and upper chest. Since such tension reduces the effective lung capacity, this would, on its own, be enough to recommend the exercise to those with asthma. There are, however, a number of other significant benefits attached to these moves.

These benefits can be demonstrated by the following experiment. Try for a few moments to raise the shoulders high and hold them in this position. You will soon find a feeling of discomfort building up in the back of your neck. The natural tendency is to relieve this pressure by pushing the head forward. This is exactly what happens in real life except the process is slower. The more tense you become, the more your shoulders rise and the more you push your head forward.

When the head is pushed forward, the centre of gravity of the body comes forward. The muscles, particularly those in the lower back, must work much harder to maintain balance. The results are:

- lower back pain;
- neck pain and headaches;
- increased risk of falls and damage to knee joints;
- reduced effective lung capacity, which continues to decrease over the years as the muscles lose their fight against gravity and the posture starts to stoop more and more;
- a shift from diaphragmatic to upper chest breathing, which raises anxiety levels and reduces circulation of blood and lymph within the body torso;
- tilting downward of the head – such a posture tends to reinforce low spirits, negativity and depression.

And all this can be prevented by the simple shoulder rolling exercises in this program!

Note Rolling the shoulders separately (one at a time) helps break muscular tension that draws the shoulder blades together. Rolling the shoulder blades alternately (so that one is up while the other is down) can double this benefit, but you still need to loosen up each shoulder separately before doing the alternate shoulder rolling.

Exercise 3   Swinging Arms

CONTINUITY

From the end position of Exercise 2, shift the weight to the right foot and step out with the left foot so that the feet are now about shoulder-width and a half apart, with the toes facing to the front. No adjustment is necessary for those doing the sitting version of the exercises.

PHYSICAL MOVEMENT

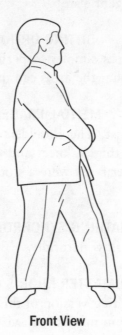

Front View

- Keeping the back straight, sink the body by feeling as though low-ered by a string attached to the crown of the head. The knees will bend naturally. While you should sink as far as comfortable, do not sink so far that the knees extend in front of the toes. (If you have been too ambitious and the position becomes uncomfortable, slowly rise up and then sink down to a comfortable height.)
- With the arms loose and relaxed at your side, bring your focus to the waist. Using the waist, turn slowly as far to the left as you comfortably can. (Do not strain, keep the body upright.) Then slowly reverse the motion and turn as far to the right as you comfortably can. Repeat turning to the left and right, slowly turn-ing faster. With the arms loose and relaxed you will find that, as you increase speed, the arms will come outwards from the waist and naturally wrap around the body. Just let this happen naturally. There is no pause between the end of one turn and the beginning of another.
- After performing the movement for about two minutes, gradually

slow the movement, turning less and less to each side until you gradually come to a gentle stop.

SITTING OPTION

If anything, this exercise is simpler to perform from a sitting position but you need to ensure that the arms can move freely.

MENTAL IMAGERY

The focus is on the waist. The shoulders and arms are relaxed and empty. The lower body, thighs, knees and feet remain in one position. It is as though your lower body were a stool that you were sitting on.

BREATHING SYNCHRONISATION

Just allow the breath to flow naturally.

GRANDMASTER KHOR'S KEY POINTS

1. When doing the standing version of this movement, one way to avoid the very common mistake of twisting through the knees is to use the 'horse-riding' position. However, one mistake should not be replaced by another, so it is important that the spine remains upright and extended throughout the move. To ensure that you sink down without spoiling your posture, revert to the image of being supported by a string through the crown of the head and feeling yourself lowered from above. As you sink down into the horse-riding position, visualise yourself as pressing the thighs against the horse. The shape made by your legs is then more of a 'u' shape rather than a 'v' shape.

2. Make sure that the body turns through the waist rather than through the knees. Turning the body by twisting the knees not only has no benefit, but may damage the knees. One of the advantages of the horse-riding position is that it helps reduce movement in the knees.

3. Ensure that the spine remains upright and rotates on its axis rather than twisting from side to side. You can tell whether or not this is happening by visualising that your eyes are painting an imaginary line around the room. The line should be the same height from the

floor throughout the whole move. Another indication of a twisting rather than rotating spine is seeing a lot of floor, especially at the end of the turns.

4. Keep all tension out of the arms and shoulders.
5. Do not stop suddenly at the end of the movement or you will tense the abdominal area.

BENEFITS

Just as aggressive stress-based tension tends to get stored in the shoulder area so emotionally based tensions tend to get stored in the abdomen. The fact that you might not show or feel a lot of emotion usually means that the abdomen has more stored tension rather than less!

When the abdomen is tense, the lung diaphragm can have a lot of difficulty moving downwards. This decreases the effective lung capacity by as much as a third. The faster breathing that becomes necessary raises anxiety and stress levels. The rigidity in the abdominal area can also interfere with digestion.

Exercise 4 Abdominal Massage

CONTINUITY

If you are uncomfortable in the horse-riding position, you can transfer the weight back to the right foot and bring the left foot inwards so that the feet are shoulder-width apart, toes pointing to the front. The knees remain off-lock. If you are comfortable in the horse-riding position, no change is necessary. For the sitting position, no change is necessary.

WARNING
While this movement is generally quite safe, medical advice should be taken if you have had any recent surgery or if surgery is planned for conditions such as a rumbling appendix or a bowel problem. The movement is also contraindicated for pregnancy. If there is any pain when performing this movement, lighten the pressure and if pain persists, cease massaging and seek medical advice before resuming the exercise.

PHYSICAL MOVEMENT

- Place the palm of the left hand on the abdomen so that your palm rests just inside of the right pelvic bone. Place the right hand over your left. Keep the shoulders relaxed.

  The abdominal area remains covered during the movement but it will obviously be easier to perform the exercise in something like a t-shirt. The more layers of clothing that you have and the more buttons, pockets and so forth that can get in the way, the more difficult it will be to perform this movement satisfactorily.

- Press down GENTLY as you move the hands upwards to just under the rib cage. Still pressing gently, pull the hands across the top of the abdomen just under the rib cage. Then push the hands downward along the left side of the abdomen to just inside the pelvic bone. Then pull them across to the right hip where you started.
- Repeat the circling of the abdominal area at least 36 times.
- Finish by bringing the hands just under the navel (see picture above).

SITTING OPTION

Again, as long as the back is upright with a feeling of suspension from the crown of the head, the movement can be performed in the sitting position as easily as in the standing position.

MENTAL IMAGERY

Imagine there is a beam of energy extending into the abdomen from your left palm that is moving and stirring the contents of your abdomen. While this is a massage movement, it is still a '*chi* massage movement'. This means that the mental focus is much more important than the pressure applied.

BREATHING SYNCHRONISATION

Match the movement of your hands to the breathing pattern. Breathe in as you move the hands upwards and across to your left side. Breathe out as you bring the hands downward and across to your right side.

GRANDMASTER KHOR'S KEY POINTS

1. Always move in the directions given above. This follows the natural movement of the digestive process along the ascending, transverse and descending colon.
2. Use a gentle but firm pressure.
3. Avoid this exercise if you have just eaten a large meal or are having abdominal problems.

BENEFITS

In terms of asthma, the direct benefits are related to the loosening up of the abdominal cavity and the release of tensions held within the musculature and internal organs. This allows the lung diaphragm to move freely, and deep, slow diaphragmatic breathing can take place.

Outside of direct effects on asthma, this exercise is one of the most popular Chinese exercises because of the general health benefits that occur when the exercise is performed regularly. The movement tones the functioning of the digestive system and results in a feeling of vitality and ease.

Exercise 5 Breathing Visualisations

Now that the stresses and tensions that might interfere with the breathing process have been eliminated, it is appropriate to focus on the breathing process itself.

CONTINUITY

From the last exercise your hands should be resting against the abdomen, one on top of the other, just below the navel.

PHYSICAL MOVEMENT

There are no physical movements involved but before commencing the visualisations re-check that:

- the body hangs as though suspended from the crown of the head;
- the tailbone is tucked under and the knees off-lock;
- the mouth is gently closed, the tongue resting against the back of the upper set of teeth, the teeth slightly separated and the jaw relaxed;

- the shoulders are relaxed.

Then slowly close your eyes and carry out the mental visualisations detailed below.

MENTAL IMAGERY

There are three parts in this breathing visualisation sequence:

1. STREAM BREATHING IMAGERY;
2. GOLDEN CLOUD BREATHING IMAGERY; and
3. THE LUNG SMILE IMAGERY.

1. STREAM BREATHING IMAGERY

- Focus on the breath, moving from the tip of the nose through the nasal passages down the throat and deep into the lungs and then up and out again. In this you are only an observer, trying to detect the physical sensations of the movement of air through the body. Do not consciously control the breath.
- Focus for a few breaths on allowing the breath to become as quiet and smooth as the body would like, then form the mental image of the air flowing down in the body to the point three finger-widths below the navel. As you do this, you will tend to find that the lung diaphragm starts to move more freely. This will be evidenced by

the feeling of the abdomen pressing outwards against the hands as you breathe in, and drawing inwards as you breathe out.

Count a dozen breaths taken in this manner.

2. GOLDEN CLOUD BREATHING IMAGERY
*   For the second part of the sequence, visualise that you are standing in the midst of a golden, glowing cloud on your in-breath — you can mentally picture this cloud being drawn deep into the lungs. Visualise the cloud inside the body as feeling warm, tingling and energising, spreading health through your body. With each in-breath, feel the warmth and light spreading first through your lungs, then through the chest, then down into the abdomen and finally throughout the limbs.

Count a dozen breaths taken in this manner.

3. THE LUNG SMILE IMAGERY
*   Imagine yourself smiling. This is a state of mind rather than the physical upturning of the mouth. (It can be useful to have an image of some event involving family, pets or friends that creates this feeling of smiling when you think of it.) Visualise your lungs as two areas of glowing whiteness and as you breathe into and out of this area imagine yourself directing your smile internally to your lungs.

Count a dozen breaths taken in this manner.

GRANDMASTER KHOR'S KEY POINTS FOR BREATHING VISUALISATIONS

You may gain more benefit by attending to the following points during the breathing visualisations:

1. Do not over-inflate or over-empty the lungs. You can tell when you are doing this because there will be a feeling of tension in the upper chest when you breathe too much air in and tension just under the rib cage when you are breathing too much air out.

2. Make the change from in-breath to out-breath and from out-breath to in-breath smooth and flowing. If it helps, visualise a candle flame an inch or so from your nostrils and imagine yourself breathing in a manner that does not cause the candle to flicker.

3. Make sure you have the sense of the crown of the head being lifted upwards and the rest of the body simply hanging from this point. The Chinese refer to the sensation created as 'riding the wind'.

BENEFITS

1. STREAM BREATHING IMAGERY

This visualisation helps to activate the lung diaphragm. This in turn means less frequent, deeper breaths that reduce anxiety and initiate the relaxation response. The effective capacity of the lungs is also substantially increased.

There is also some interesting energy work going on. *Chi* energy is not only stimulated by needles, pressure and massage but by mental focus and placement. In this exercise, the centre of the palm will be over the *tan tien* area, three-finger widths below the navel. (This brings the *lao gong* acupoint on the palm over the *chi hai* acupoint on the *ren mai* meridian. This has benefits because the *chi hai* point is a major controlling point for the efficiency of the respiratory function. Also, the *lao gong* point is a major point for projecting *chi* to open up or reinforce the energy of other acupoints.) This may be one reason why focus on the *chi hai* point seems to induce increased movement in the lung diaphragm.

2. GOLDEN CLOUD BREATHING IMAGERY

This is an energising breath that both encourages the flow of *chi* throughout the body and helps to maintain a state of deep relaxation.

3. THE LUNG SMILE IMAGERY

Smiling is often misunderstood as being the movement of the mouth. In fact smiling is a state of mind, and one of its physical expressions is the upturned mouth. There are, however, many other things going on as well. X-ray photography of the bodies of people before and during a smile shows dramatic differences in the degree of tensions held within the internal organs. When you direct a smile at an internal organ, you are directing blood and energy to that organ, and removing stress and tension. The organ will be much better for it.

The visualisation of the colour white is related to the fact that energy comes in wavelengths. When we mentally visualise white, we are also generating the wavelength of *chi* that most closely corresponds to the lung's *chi* energy. Sound also has wavelengths and was used in Chinese Taoist healing practices. The sound that reinforces the lung energy is a 'sssss' sound and it is effective in this visualisation to breathe out through the mouth making a continuous 'sssss' sound.

Exercise 6   Supplementary Optional Exercises

HOW TO USE THE SUPPLEMENTARY EXERCISE SET

All of the exercises in this group will be of particular use to those with asthma. However, if you are keeping to the 30-minute program time, it will generally preclude you from performing more than one of these exercises in each exercise session. There is, of course, no reason why you should not extend the program past the 30-minute limit by including more than one of these exercises. Other alternatives are to use different exercises on different days. This will also help to keep novelty and interest in the program.

The three exercises chosen are the The Taoist Archer, The Heavenly Lift, and The Buddha Smelling Roses. All these exercises can be modified to be performed from the sitting position.

CONTINUITY

The Taoist Archer and Buddha Smelling Roses exercises are performed with the shoulder-and-a-half width stance, and if moving from the previous exercise or from the Heavenly lift exercise, it will be necessary to step out to this stance. Otherwise no adjustments are necessary.

With the sitting form of the exercises, no adjustments are necessary.

Supplementary Exercise 2 — The Taoist Archer

PHYSICAL MOVEMENTS

The Taoist Archer is a quite complex movement. To make it easier to learn, it has been broken up into a number of parts. It is recommended that you practise each part until you are familiar with it before going on to the next part.

If you are using the sitting movements then simply follow the arm-work instructions and ignore the legwork, and the sinking and rising movements.

SWORDFINGERS HAND POSITION

Before practising the Taoist Archer movement itself, you should be familiar with the swordfingers hand position that is used in the movement.

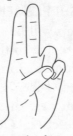

Extend the first two fingers directly forward while curling the third and fourth fingers so that the back of the last segment of each of these fingers can rest against the inside of the last segment of the thumb. The top of the thumbnail should be more or less aligned with the top crease of these fingers.

Check:

- The first and second fingers are straight.
- The thumb, palm, third and fourth fingers form as large a circle as is comfortable.

TAOIST ARCHER MOVEMENT SEQUENCE

PREPARATION — PART ONE

From a shoulder-width and a half stance:

- Arc the hands upwards and forwards to chest height. The arms are extended in front of the body. The palms face down and fingertips point forward.

  Make sure that the arms remain relaxed as they are extended. There should be no straightening of the elbows or lifting of the shoulders. If the wrists are not brought above shoulder height and the elbows remain lower than shoulders and wrists, then the weight of the arm pulls the shoulder joint down.

- Now, imagining yourself suspended from the crown of your head. Feel yourself being slowly lowered down, your knees bending and your back remaining straight. At the same time, draw the elbows slowly down towards the sides of the body so that the hands arc downwards to finish at the sides of the body. Palms face to the rear. The fingertips point downwards.

  Make sure that the back remains straight.

MOVEMENT FIRING BOW TO LEFT SIDE – PART ONE

OVERVIEW
Visualise the right hand holding an arrow and bowstring and the left hand holding the bow. Place the arrow to the bow, stretch the bow to full extension and release the arrow to its target. Then return the bow to your side.

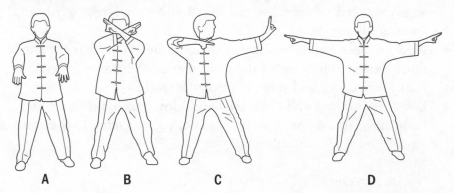

A   B   C   D

- Arc the hands upwards and forwards to chest height, extended in front of the body. Palms face down, fingertips point forward. Elbows and shoulders are relaxed.
- Lower and draw in the elbows, bringing the arms in to cross at the wrists at heart height in front of the centre-line of the body. Make sure that the armpits and elbow joints remain open and relaxed. The back of the left wrist rests against the front of the right wrist. At the same time, form each hand into the swordfingers position (see explanation above).
- Rotate the left wrist outwards and push the left hand to the left so that the left arm is extended from the left side of the body, the left hand at shoulder height. The swordfingers of the left hand point upwards. The left palm faces outwards from the left side.

  At the same time, draw the right elbow to the right so that it finishes at shoulder height in a direct line with the shoulders. The right hand is at chest height, the palm facing the body, the sword fingers pointing to the left. The crease of the right wrist should be almost opposite the right armpit.

  Also at the same time, turn the head to the left to look over the tip of the left swordfingers. (This is the direction you would be releasing the arrow in.)

  When you draw the bow, feel a full stretch across the chest but keep the shoulders down. This helps to free up contracted inter-coastal muscles that may be acting to constrict the breathing. Make sure the shoulders remain down and relaxed.
- As you mentally release the arrow, simultaneously release the swordfingers and arc the right hand backwards to finish with both arms extended to the sides, and the shoulders, elbows, wrists and hands all in one line.
- Now arc both hands forward at shoulder height so that the hands finish extended in front of the body, shoulder distance apart. Palms face down and fingertips point forward.
- Lower the elbows and draw the hands down to the sides of the body, fingertips pointing to the ground, palms facing to the rear.

MOVEMENT FIRING BOW TO RIGHT SIDE – PART TWO

OVERVIEW
Visualise the right hand holding an arrow and bowstring and the left hand holding the bow. Place the arrow to the bow, stretch the bow to full extension and release the arrow to its target. Then return the bow to your side.

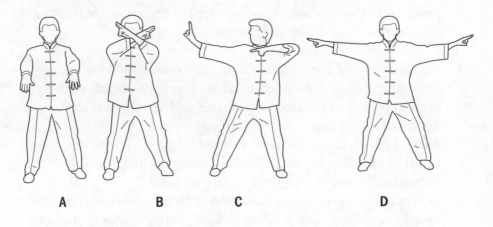

A   B   C   D

- Arc the hands upwards and forwards to chest height, extended in front of the body. Palms face down, fingertips point forward. Elbows and shoulders are relaxed.
- Lower and draw in the elbows, bringing the arms in to cross at the wrists at heart height in front of the centre-line of the body. Make sure that the armpits and elbow joints remain open and relaxed. The back of the right wrist rests against the front of the left wrist. At the same time, form each hand into the swordfingers position (see explanation above).
- Rotate the right wrist outwards and push the right hand to the right so that the right arm is extended from the right side of the body, the right hand at shoulder height. The swordfingers of the right hand point upwards. The right palm faces outwards from the right side.

At the same time, draw the left elbow to the left so that it finishes at shoulder height in a direct line with the shoulders. The left hand is at chest height, the palm facing the body, and the swordfingers pointing to the right. The crease of the left wrist should be almost opposite the left armpit.

Also at the same time, turn the head to the right to look over the tip of the right swordfingers. (This is the direction you would be releasing the arrow in.)

When you draw the bow, feel a full stretch across the chest but keep the shoulders down. This helps to free up contracted intercoastal muscles that may be acting to constrict the breathing. Make sure the shoulders remain down and relaxed.

- As you mentally release the arrow, simultaneously release the swordfingers and arc the left hand backwards to finish with both arms extended to the sides, and the shoulders, elbows, wrists and hands all in one line.
- Now arc both hands forward at shoulder height so that the hands finish extended in front of the body, shoulder distance apart. Palms face down and fingertips point forward.
- Lower the elbows and draw the hands down to the sides of the body, fingertips pointing to the ground, palms facing to the rear.

Repeat the entire movement (right and left sides) eight times.

MOVEMENT CO-ORDINATION
This is a fairly complex move so here is a simplified description.

- Step out to shoulder-width and a half stance.
- Float hands up to shoulder height, then sink as you bring hands down to side.
- Bring hands up in front and form swordfingers.
- Turn head to left as you stretch bow.
- Release arrow and take hands out to either side of shoulders.
- Turn head to face front as you bring hands forward and then down to sides.
- Bring hands up in front and form swordfingers.
- Turn head to right as you stretch bow.
- Release arrow and extend hand to either side of shoulders.

- Turn head to face front as you bring hands back in front of shoulders.
- Bring hands down to the side.

BREATHING SYNCHRONISATION

There are two breathing patterns recommended. The two breaths per movement (double breath) pattern where the practitioner has difficulty in getting the breath rate below about six breaths per minute without forcing; and the one breath movement (single breath) pattern where the practitioner can comfortably hold their breathing below six breaths per minute.

DOUBLE BREATH PATTERN

Breathe in as you bring the hands up to heart height and form sword-fingers. Breathe out as you bring the hands in to cross in front of the chest. Breathe in as you stretch the bow and breathe, and breathe out as you release the arrow and bring the hands forward and to the sides.

SINGLE BREATH PATTERN

Breathe in as you draw the bow. Breathe out as you release the arrow and take the hands to the sides.

MENTAL IMAGERY

The name of this movement is the Taoist Archer because the Taoists were noted for their sense of calmness and focus. The mental image is thus not a martial one but one of relaxed centredness.

Take the imagery seriously and you can train yourself to think confidently and positively (instead of unwittingly training oneself to think uncertainly and negatively). Visualising a target and having the positivity to believe that even mentally you can see the arrow fly direct to the target is one way of exercising yourself to think positively.

One study on positive thinking was done on basketball players. One group was put through additional standard physical training. The other group merely spent the same amount of time visualising themselves being successful with their various basketball shots. Both groups were found to have improved equally!

Some people's thoughts may be programmed so that they have

difficulty even in making the positive visualisation of a successful archery shot. We can borrow a visualisation from the ancient archers to remedy this. When they were ready to shoot, the archers would imagine that the arrow grew longer until the point extended to touch the centre of the target. Once this had been achieved, the archer then let go of the tail of the arrow. Obviously they could not miss because the arrow had already reached the target.

This is similar to the positive thinking techniques of today where we visualise, not the image of where we want to go, but the image that we have arrived or completed the activity.

GRANDMASTER KHOR'S KEY POINTS

1. Do not overfill or over-empty the lungs so that you feel strain and tension.
2. Keep the shoulders relaxed.
3. Feel the stretch before releasing the arrow.
4. Stretch gently, do not force – the stretch will build up over time.
5. The eyes look directly where you are mentally targetting the arrow.
6. Keep the back straight at all times.

BENEFITS

This exercise has a number of benefits for people with asthma:

- It expands the lung cage with the stretches, reducing stress and tension in the intercoastal muscles.
- It encourages deep diaphragmatic breathing.
- The action of the movement stimulates a neural plexus under the sternum that helps stimulate the immune and defensive system.
- The movement strengthens positive attitude and approach to life, increasing willpower and determination.

Supplementary Exercise 2 – The Heavenly Lift

WARNING
In cases of high blood pressure, pregnancy, abdominal conditions such as hernia, or recent surgery, seek medical advice before stretching the hands upward over the head. (An alternative is to make the arm stretch horizontally in front of the body rather than over the head.)

PHYSICAL MOVEMENT — Part One

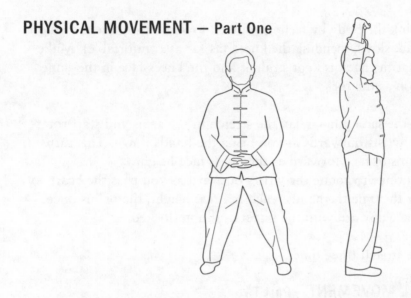

- Commence from a standing position with feet parallel and shoulder-width apart. The knees are off-lock. The hands are brought together in front of the *tan tien*, fingers interlocked. The palms face up.

  Hold the interlocked palms 10 centimetres or so in front of the body. This prevents cutting the circulation at the elbows and putting tension in the shoulders when you lift the hands.

- Imagine yourself as though supported by a string from the crown of the head, then visualise yourself being drawn upwards from this point until the legs are straight.

    At the same time, lift the palms (fingers still interlocked)

91

upwards in front of the centre-line of the body and extend them over the head.

As the hands rise up past the heart, rotate the wrists so the palms face the heart point.
As the hands pass the heart, start to rotate them outwards so that the palms face forward.
As the palms are taken over the head, turn the palms to face upwards and straighten the arms in a stretch.

- Now sink the body by feeling yourself lowered from the crown of the head, slowly bending the knees (as far as comfortable). Make sure that the back is kept straight and the knees face in the same direction as the toes.

    At the same time, relax the stretch in the arms and start rotating the wrists outwards as you bring the hands down. This turns the palms to face forward as they pass face height.

    Continue to rotate the wrists outward as you pass the heart so that by the time the hands reach *tan tien* height, the palms once more face upward with the fingers still interlocked.

Repeat the stretch three times.

PHYSICAL MOVEMENT —Part Two

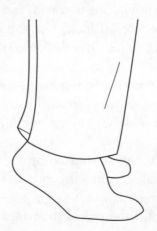

This part of the movement is exactly the same as in Part One except that:

- In the upward part of the movement, once you have straightened the legs, you continue moving up by lifting the heels slightly off the ground so that the body is supported on the ball of the toes of both feet.

  It is important to keep the body upright without leaning forward or backward. Do not come up on the tips of the toes.

  In the downward part of the movement as you start to sink the body, first lower the heels gently, and slowly, to the ground. Once the heels are on the ground continue, as in Part One, to lower the body by bending the knees as far as comfortable.

  Make sure that the back stays straight throughout the movement and the knees face in the same direction as the toes. If you force too far down, the knees will either turn inwards towards each other or outwards away from each other.

Repeat this movement eight times.

SITTING VARIATION

Follow the instructions that relate to armwork but ignore those that relate to legwork and sinking and rising.

BREATHING SYNCHRONISATION

There are two breathing patterns recommended: the 'double breathspattern', where the practitioner has difficulty in getting the breath rate below about six breaths per minute without forcing; and the 'single breath pattern', where the practitioner can comfortably hold their breathing rate below about six breaths per minute.

DOUBLE BREATH PATTERN
- Breathe in as you bring the hands up to heart height.
- Breathe out as you extend the hands upward.

- Breathe in as you bring the hands down to heart height.
- Breathe out as you take the hands down to *tan tien*.

SINGLE BREATH PATTERN
- Breathe in on the upward stretch as you rise.
- Breathe out on the downward movement as you sink.

MENTAL IMAGERY

To get the full benefits of the movement, it is important to keep the movement slow and relaxed and maintain a strong connection between the physical movement and the breathing pattern. One image you can use is to:

- As the hands move upwards, visualise the level of air rising in the lungs (as though they were filling up with a fluid rather than air).
- As the hands move downwards, visualise the level of air sinking in the lungs (as though the air was fluid draining out of the lungs).

GRANDMASTER KHOR'S KEY POINTS

1. Keep the back straight at all times.
2. Do not overfill the lungs. Keep them relaxed by breathing in to about 75 per cent capacity.
3. Move slowly, lowering the heels gently to the ground. Make very sure you do not drop the heels to the ground with the knees locked.
4. Extend the hands vertically above the *bai huai* point in the centre of the top of the skull. If the hands are forward, this may throw you off balance.
5. Stretch gently. Do not force. The stretch will build up naturally as you repeat the movement.
6. The eyes look directly forward throughout the movement.
7. Do not lean forward when you bend the knees.

BENEFITS

The exercise works on the triple heater meridian that balances the *chi* energy in the major areas of the body. In terms of asthma, such balancing can improve the energy available in the thoracic cavity that supports the respiration function. The nature of the movement also slows down the breathing, helping to induce the relaxation response.

Supplementary Exercise 3 — Buddha Smelling Roses

PHYSICAL MOVEMENTS

From the Quiet Standing/Sitting position.

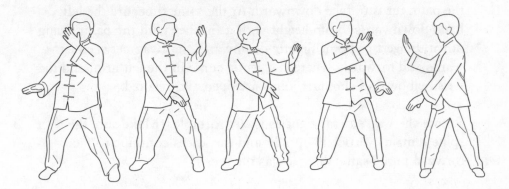

- Bend the knees and sink down into the 'horse-riding' position.

- Bring the left hand up in front of the centre-line of the body. The palm faces the body at about throat height. The fingers of the left hand point to the right and upwards. The left arm is gently curved with the wrist, elbow joint and shoulders open and relaxed.

    At the same time, take the right hand down so that it is at hip height and extended outwards from the right hip. The right palm faces down, fingertips point outwards and halfway between right-wards and forwards. There is a gentle curve in the right arm, and the wrist, elbow and shoulder joints are open and relaxed.

Look forwards into the distance over the tips of the left fingers.

- Rotate the waist as far left as is comfortable. (Make sure the spine remains vertically upright and the knees continue to face forward in the same direction as the toes.)

It is the turning of the body that makes the arms appear to move. Do not move the arms independently or you will close them against the body, causing tension in the shoulders. The left hand will thus remain in front of the centre-line of the body while the right is out in front of the right hip. Throughout the turn, keep the eyes looking out over the tip of the left fingers

- As you reach the limit of the turn, rotate the left wrist inwards until the palm turns to face downward. At the same time, arc the left hand downwards to hip height until it finishes with the palm facing down. Fingertips point slightly downwards, halfway between left-wards and forwards. There is a gentle curve in the left arm, and the wrist, elbow and shoulder joints are open and relaxed.

- Rotate the waist as far right as is comfortable. (Make sure the spine remains vertically upright and the knees continue to face forward in the same direction as the toes.)

The body brings the arms around with it. Do not move your arms independently. The right hand will thus remain in front of the centre-line of the body while the left is out in front of the left hip. Throughout the turn, keep the eyes looking out over the tip of the right fingers.

- As you reach the limit of the turn, rotate the right wrist inwards until the palm turns to face downwards. At the same time, arc the right hand downwards to hip height until it finishes with the palm facing down. Fingertips point slightly downwards, halfway between rightwards and forwards. There is a gentle curve in the right arm, and the wrist, elbow and shoulder joints are open and relaxed.

  At the same time, rotate the left wrist outwards until the palm turns to face the body and arc the left hand upwards to throat height, palm facing the body.

Fingertips point halfway between upwards and rightwards.

Repeat the entire movement eight times.

Then relax hands down to the side and straighten knees to off-lock position.

BREATHING SYNCHRONISATION

- Breathe in as you raise the left hand and make the half turn to the left.
- Breathe out as you sink the left hand.
- Breathe in as you make the full turn to the left.
- Breathe out as you sink the right hand.
- Breathe in as you make the full turn to the right.
- On closing, breathe out as you relax both hands down to the sides.
- Breathe in as you straighten the knees.

MENTAL IMAGERY

Imagine that the palm raised in front of you is carrying a rose (or if you are allergic to roses, any other fragrant flower), and try to smell the fragrance.

One way to do this exercise is to rub lavender oil into the palms before doing the exercise. Lavender is one of those smells that induce the relaxation response. Other aromas that can be beneficial for asthmatics are mentioned in Part 4.

As a general rule, it is not a bad idea to make sure that when you exercise, it is in the presence of beneficial aromas. Using essential oils on the hands or skin not only keeps you close to the aroma, but the body heat helps to volatilise the oil and there is absorption of the beneficial properties directly through the skin. Naturally, if you have asthma attacks that are allergy-triggered, do not use any aromas or oils that you may be sensitive too.

GRANDMASTER KHOR'S KEY POINTS

1. Keep the spine upright.
2. Keep the weight equally centred on both feet.

3. Do not twist through the knees.
4. Keep the fingers extended but not stretched.

The repositioning of hands that occurs at the end of each turn should be done slowly so that the time taken to exchange the hands is the same as the time taken to turn from side to side. This allows the in-breath and out-breath to remain balanced.

BENEFITS

Activates the *su liao* acupoint on the tip of the nose. This improves the respiration function. The movement of the arms is also good for stimulating energy flow along the lung meridian and this is a very good exercise for the diaphragm because of the combined effect of turning of the waist with the deep diaphragmatic breathing. The movement also helps to reduce rigidity and congestion in the abdominal area and stimulates the digestive function. This movement is particularly good for initiating the relaxation response.

Exercise 7 Opening the Chest

CONTINUITY

Depending on the supplementary exercise that you finished on, you may need to step back into the shoulder-width stance before continuing with the opening the chest movement.

PHYSICAL MOVEMENT

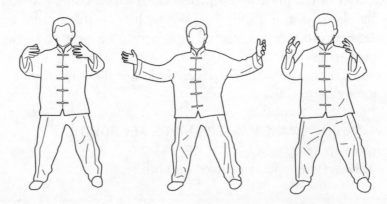

- Let both hands drift forward and upward until they reach shoulder height in front of the body. The palms face down and the fingertips are extended gently forward. At the same time as you do this, imagine yourself drawn upward from the crown of the head causing the knees to slowly straighten.

  Make sure that the elbows and shoulders remain relaxed, the elbows being slightly below shoulder height.

- Rotate the wrists inwards so that the palms face each other, then draw out the hands to the sides as far as is comfortable. Palms face to the front.

  Again it is important to make sure that the elbow and shoulder joints remain relaxed, and that the elbows are lower than the shoulders. The wrists are also relaxed so the fingertips face forwards on an angle. Without causing discomfort, you should bring the arms far enough to the sides to feel a stretch occurring through the rib cage.

- Reverse the motion above, bringing the hands back in front of the body, palms facing each other at shoulder height. The arms are gently extended, not stretched.
- Rotate the wrists to turn the palms down then draw the elbows down, pushing downwards with the palms as they come back to the side of the body. At the same time as you do this, feel your body lowered from the crown of the head so that the knees slowly bend. You should now be in the same position as you started.

Repeat the entire movement at least eight times.

BREATHING SYNCHRONISATION

- Breathe in as you lift the arms up and take them out to the sides.
- Breathe out as you bring the arms back in front of the body and lower them to the sides.

MENTAL IMAGERY

Imagine that you are standing in the ocean and that your hands are slowly floating to the surface. No effort is required on the upward movement. As you open your hands to the side, smile internally and look forward into the distance. As you sink the hands down to the side again, imagine that you are standing in the ocean and that you have to gently push your hands down through the water.

GRANDMASTER KHOR'S KEY POINTS

1. Keep the spine straight and the shoulders relaxed. Take particular care in this as you bring the arms outwards to the sides.
2. Perform the movement at a speed that comfortably matches your breathing pattern. Go as slow as you can but not so slow that you run out of breath or overfill the lungs and end up feeling tense and strained.
3. Do not straighten elbow joints.

BENEFITS

Increases the oxygen supply to the cerebrum, resulting in clearer thinking and increased awareness. This creates a feeling of expansiveness, joy and confidence. The movement also acts to expand the ribcage and enhance the relaxation response.

Exercise 8 Lung Meridian Acupressure Massage

CONTINUITY

Maintain the stance you were in at the end of the opening the chest movement.

PHYSICAL MOVEMENT

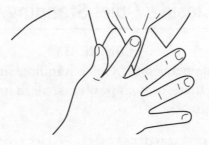

1. Place the index finger of one hand gently on the suprasternal by the meeting of the bones just below the base of the throat. Take three deep breaths and relax.
2. Using the pad of the right thumb, massage the fleshy pad under the left thumb (from lower thumb joint to wrist) for about 30 seconds. Repeat process on other hand.
3. Place the right palm over the back of the left wrist and lightly wrap the fingers and thumb around the left wrist. Rotate the left hand back and forwards to massage the left wrist 36 times. Now with the right thumb and fingers still wrapped around the left wrist, push the right hand up and down between the crease of the elbow and wrist 36 times. Repeat process on other hand.

MENTAL IMAGERY

Keep your mind focused on what you are doing. Use the mind rather than physical force. All movements should be slow and deliberate.

BREATHING SYNCHRONISATION

Take care to maintain the relaxed breathing pattern while performing the massage.

BENEFITS

The lung meridian runs along the arms and thumbs and this massage sequence covers the main points in those areas that are involved with asthma.

Massage in these areas will help maintain a proper flow of *chi* along the lung meridian that will help to support the lung function.

Exercise 9   Closing: Quiet Standing/Sitting

CONTINUITY

You should have maintained the Quiet Standing/Sitting while performing the massage so that, for both positions, all that it is necessary to do is recheck the key points.

PHYSICAL MOVEMENT – QUIET STANDING

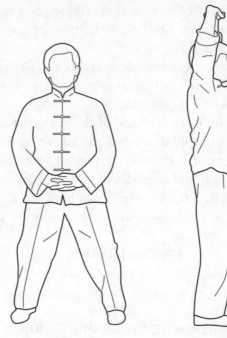

Front View   **Side View**

KEY POINTS TO RECHECK

- Your feet are shoulder-width apart. The feet parallel with the toes pointing to the front.

  Refocus on how the feet are carrying the body weight. Try to feel as though the weight is equally distributed between both feet and centred between the toes and heels. If the weight comes forward on the toes, backward onto the heels or sideways onto one foot or the other, it will cause muscular tension and postural distortion. Check that your toes just rest gently on the ground and are not clenched or upturned.

- Your body is as though supported by a string attached to the crown of your head. Your whole body can hang down from this point with the weight of your body supported by the string. Your knees are in the off-lock position.
- The pelvis is relaxed. The arms hang loosely by the sides.
- The mouth is gently closed, the tip of the tongue resting against the back of the upper set of teeth, or on the hard palate if this is comfortable.
- You are breathing through the nose, relaxed and natural.

When you have completed this check, bring the hands inwards over the abdomen so that the right palm rests on the surface of the abdomen just below the navel and the left palm is placed over the back of the right hand palm and close with 12 relaxed breaths.

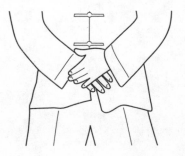

MENTAL IMAGERY AND BREATHING SYNCHRONISATION

Remember, do not control your breaths; just be aware of your body breathing and count each in-breath and out-breath as it happens. If you watch your breathing, you will find that it almost naturally slows, and as it slows, you become more relaxed.

BENEFITS

The major benefits of practising the Quiet Standing/Sitting at the end of the session are that you should finish as relaxed and focused as possible so that you can take that relaxation and focus with you into your daily routine. It is also an opportunity to compare just how relaxed you feel at the end of the session to the beginning. However, do understand that the first few times you perform this session you will have the 'stress' of learning the movements to contend with. Once you have performed the session about half a dozen times, you will really begin to appreciate just how relaxed the program can make you.

PART 4

Additional Body–Mind Techniques for Asthma Management

THIS PART OF THE BOOK contains a number of additional body–mind medicine techniques that are useful from an asthma perspective especially. These techniques can be performed before or after or be completely independent from the exercise session detailed in Part 3 of this book. These techniques can be grouped under the following headings:

1. Additional breathing technique
2. Additional acumassage techniques
3. Lung reflexology techniques
4. Moxabustion techniques
5. Positive thinking techniques
6. Feng Shui techniques
7. Body–mind aspects of nutrition

1. ADDITIONAL BREATHING TECHNIQUE

The cleansing breath

The purity of the air within the lungs is particularly important to asthmatics and they should always seek to ensure that the quality of the air that they breathe is as high as possible. Every now and then, however, exposure to smoky, polluted air may occur. This can tend to sit in the lungs for long periods of time, especially when sleeping. It is therefore good that once the smoky or polluted air has been left behind, we seek to expel any contaminated residue that remains in the lungs.

From the Quiet Standing/Sitting position, allow your breath to settle and slow. Then place your palms just under the rib cage, fingers pointing towards one another. As you breathe out, bend forward from the waist and press gently inwards and upwards with the palms of your hands, making a conscious effort to expel all the air that you can. On the in-breath, you release the pressure of the hand and straighten up. The exercise is performed three times only. Then do Quiet Standing/Sitting again and allow the breath to normalise.

This is the one instance when we breathe out through the mouth. The in-breath is still done through the nose.

> **WARNING**
> *The cleansing breath has been included here because there are specific situations in which it may be very useful to asthmatics. However, it does involve 'forced' breathing and should be used cautiously by asthmatics to ensure that they are not one of those rare cases where performing this exercise may trigger an asthmatic attack.*

Try to maintain softness, quietness and fluidity of breathing while performing the cleansing breath. Your breathing before and after should be in and out through the nose.

2. ADDITIONAL ACUMASSAGE TECHNIQUES

Working on the lung meridian

Space does not permit a detailed explanation of the *chi* energy meridian system and the way it functions but to enable the person with asthma to take advantage of some additional techniques that can strengthen the lung meridian, some basic information on the meridian system and how it operates is provided below.

The relationship of chi to the meridians

Chi is much more than bio-electricity or bio-magnetism but these provide us with a useful concept for visualising *chi*. *Chi* is the life energy that flows not only within us but between the environment and the body.

We obtain *chi* from the air we breathe, the water we drink, the food we eat and the environment that we live in. We expend *chi* in our mental and physical activities – keeping our bodies running, thinking, generating emotion, working and playing.

Like electricity, *chi* flows in currents but also creates fields. The body thus has a *chi* field and the *chi* itself flows along pathways in the body known as meridians. These meridians exist on an energetic rather than physical level but they can still be verified by measuring changes in the electro-potential of the skin, that is, the ability of the skin to conduct electricity along the body. This is very prevalent in acupoints, which are simply areas where the flow of the *chi* energy can be influenced from the surface of the body by acupressure, acumassage and moxabustion.

The geography of the lung meridian

The lung meridian is one of 12 organ meridians. It travels in the pathway outlined in the diagram below.

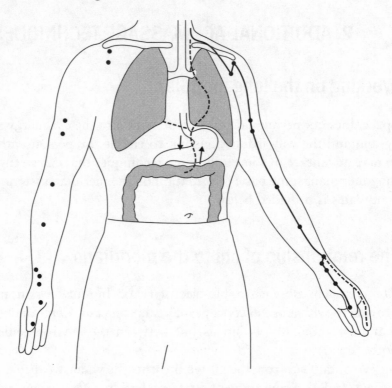

Meridians are always paired and the meridian paired with the lung is the large intestine meridian. Since the energy of the body is one interconnected structure, all points on all meridians will have some degree of influence on every aspect of the body, but keeping the energy and function of these two meridians and organs working properly will have the most beneficial influence on asthma.

The linkage of lung and large intestine is also another reason for the importance of the abdominal massage recommended as part of the model exercise program.

Lung energy flows internally up the centre-line of the body to just behind the suprasternal notch. The *chi* flow then separates and moves outwards to the shoulders where it reaches the surface to flow downwards along the inside of the arms and up through the outer edge of the thumbs. The key acupoint on the lung meridian for asthma is called *yun men*.

KEY DETAILS FOR ACUPOINT *YUN MEN*

MEANING
Yun means cloud. *Men* means gate.

LOCATION
Just under the clavicle (or collarbone) where the clavicle connects with the shoulder.

INDICATIONS
Cough, asthma, fullness of chest.

COMMENTARY
A major point lying on the lung meridian. It is the entry point of the *chi* into the lung meridian, hence the reference to gate. It is believed to be the chief connection point for the lung meridian to Earth Chi.

Tapping this point can help to clear the lungs.

Meridian brushing

A supplementary technique that you might like to play with is meridian brushing. The aim of this technique is to stimulate the flow of *chi* along the lung meridian. This is done by either brushing the fingertips along the pathway of the meridian or moving one's mental focus along the meridian. In meridian brushing, one first condenses and relaxes *chi* by moving the hand or mind in the opposite direction to the natural flow of *chi* energy. Then one encourages the flow of the now calm, undisturbed *chi* by moving the hand or mental focus in the same direction as the natural *chi* flow.

Following the path of the lung meridian in either direction should take 20 to 30 seconds.

• Brush over the line of the lung meridian from the left thumb to about halfway between navel and sternum with the pads of the first and second fingers of the right hand. Repeat three times.
• Brush over the line of the lung meridian about halfway between navel and sternum to the left thumb, with the pads of the first and second fingers of the right hand. Repeat three times.
• Brush over the line of the lung meridian from the right thumb to about halfway between navel and sternum with the pads of the first and second fingers of the left hand. Repeat three times.
• Brush over the line of the lung meridian about halfway between navel and sternum to the right thumb with the pads of the first and second fingers of the left hand. Repeat three times.

Lung meridian acupressure massage

The lung meridian runs down the arm and terminates in the thumb. Perform the following gentle massage on yourself or use the technique on a person who has asthma. It is a good massage to perform at any time but particularly when you feel an asthma attack coming on.

STEP 1
Take the thumb of your left hand between the pads of the thumb and first finger of your right hand. Now 'roll' these around the left thumb, from its base to its tip. Use just enough tension to move the flesh of the left thumb gently backwards and forwards. As you pass the base of the

nail of the left thumb, press firmly with the right thumb and finger in a pinching motion (it should not be hard enough to cause pain), then with a slight 'flicking' motion release the pinch outwards from the tip of the thumb. Repeat this motion at least six times on the left thumb. Then change hands and perform the same massage on the right thumb.

Make sure that the pulling pressure applied is gentle. On no account should there be any excessive strain on the joints of the digit.

STEP 2

Locate the *hegu* point in the intersection of the thumb and first finger bone. An easy way to find this point is to bring the thumb and finger together. Place the pad (not nail) of the other thumb on the highest point of the mound of flesh that was created by bringing the thumb and finger together. Press downwards and under the bone of the first finger. Not too hard because the point can often be tender. If you don't think you have found the point, you haven't – you will know when you do, just continue pressing gently in a widening circle and you will find it. This point is particularly good for raising the energy and vitality of the body and was one of the key points of the ancient Taoists.

When you have found the point, with the other thumb, massage in circles slowly and firmly at least 36 times and then repeat on the other hand.

STEP 3

Press the pad of one thumb against the centre of the fleshy tissue that extends from the base of the thumb to the wrist and massage the area vigorously in circles, again a minimum of 36 times. This point may be very tender if the lung energy is disturbed and you are feeling a little depressed. Repeat on opposite side.

3. LUNG REFLEXOLOGY TECHNIQUES

There are also a number of reflexology zones on the foot, hand, ear and abdomen that are beneficial to asthma. You can use these techniques in conjunction with lung meridian acumassage. You can sometimes better understand how and why reflexology zones work by thinking of the body as having a holographic nature.

'Holographic' or reflexology zones

These zones are based on the recognition that the energy pattern of the body is holographic in nature. That is, the overall pattern of the body is held in every part. If you cut a hologram in two, you do not get one hologram of one side of the 'image' and another hologram of the other side of the 'image'. You get two 'degraded' images of the same thing. (We are talking here of laser-actuated holograms where the hologram is created by directing a laser beam onto the surface of a hologram. The cheap strips and discs that appear to create a holographic image in normal light are not true holograms and cutting these in two will not create two degraded images.) Magnets are another familiar item that demonstrates a holographic nature. Indeed some physicists speculate that the entire nature of the universe is holographic. This would certainly fit with the Chinese theories of *chi*. Be that as it may, it is certain that these 'holographic zones' can have a powerful effect on their related organs and if you have asthma it is recommended that you massage these areas.

Note The abdominal massage in the model exercise set covers the lung massage points on the abdomen, so no separate exercise is necessary.

- On the ear, the area concerned with the lungs is fairly awkward to work on. The best technique is to rest the fingertips just above the ear and reach under the earlobe with the pad of the thumb. You should then massage vigorously but gently along the hard cartilage that separates the skull from the flap of the ear.

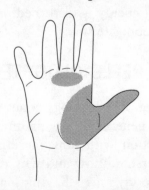

Lung reflexology zones on the hands

- On the palm side of the hands, the lung reflexology zone is in the fleshy pad that runs under the base of the fingers from about the centre of the first finger to the centre of the third finger. Massage this area.

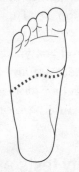

Lung reflexology zone on feet

- On the soles of the feet, the lung reflexology zone is in the fleshy pad that runs under the base of the toes from toe two to five. The lung diaphragm reflex zone runs across the foot, a line that separates the ball of the foot from the inner sole. The vertical band between the first and second toes extending across the ball of the foot is a good place to work on the trachea and bronchi. Therefore, massage the whole area under the toes that covers the ball of the foot.

- Focus on any tender areas but, as above, do not cause pain.

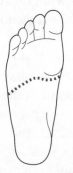

Massaging the lung diaphragm line of the foot

LUNG DIAPHRAGM LINE

- Massaging along this line improves the function of the lung diaphragm. You will probably experience a sensation of relaxation when you work here. This is because with the lung diaphragm working properly, you are taking fewer, deeper breaths and this initiates the relaxation response. This in turn increases the effective lung capacity.
- Push the pad of the thumb backwards and forwards along the lung diaphragm line. If there are any tender spots, focus on those points using a pressing circling motion. Remember this is Tai Chi massage and should not cause pain or discomfort.

Lung diapraghm activity tests and remedial massage

1. TESTING THE ACTIVITY OF THE LUNG DIAPHRAGM

The activity of the lung diaphragm is particularly subject to stress. This can build up unnoticeably over the years and considerably reduce the effective capacity of the lung. (To say nothing of the reduction of the internal massaging effect on the digestive system and internal organs.)

It was suggested earlier that if you place the left palm (fingers pointing to the right) just below the navel and the right hand over the top of the left (fingers pointing to the left), then you should be able to feel your abdomen expand with the in-breath and contract with the out-breath.

If you do not feel such movement, it is a sign of reduced activity of the lung diaphragm. Take a few moments to watch a cat, dog or baby breathe – notice that most of the movement is in the abdominal rather then chest area.

Be careful when you perform this exercise that you do not uncon-sciously sway forward on the in-breath and backward on the out-breath to create the illusion of movement in the abdomen.

One way to test for this is to leave the left hand below the navel but take the right hand behind the back and place the back of the hand (fingers pointing leftwards) over the spine at the same height as the left hand. When you breathe in, you should now feel the two hands being pushed apart. When you breath out, you should feel the hands move together.

114

2. REMEDIAL MASSAGE FOR THE LUNG DIAPHRAGM

The lung diaphragm will usually start to improve its function when you use the 'stream breathing' visualisation in the exercise program. If there remains little movement, there is a form of massage to loosen up the lung diaphragm.

Place the fingertips of the second and third fingers of each hand immediately under the rib cage on the right side of the body. The area can be quite tender and you should only use gentle pressure. Circle the fingers in a clockwise direction for about one minute (the circling should press gently up and under the rib bones). Then move the fingers two inches to the left (following the ribcage) and circle for one minute again. Continue moving and circling along the rib cage to the far left side of the body.

Remember if the area is tender to be more gentle. If you create pain, the body will tense in this area and this is the exact opposite effect of what we are trying to achieve.

The circling movements should be slow and even, and done as much with the mind as with the muscles. Keep the shoulders and fingers relaxed to aid the flow of *chi*. Use the pads of the second and third fingers to perform the massage, NOT the fingernails!

4. MOXABUSTION TECHNIQUES

MoxAbustion is the name given to the technique of burning herbs in close proximity to acupoints. The *chi* energy of the herb is then transferred into the energy meridian system. (Interestingly, studies have shown that the tissue around an acupoint builds up to a higher temperature when moxa herbs are being burned than when other heat sources of the same temperature are placed the same distance away.)

The reason that this technique has been included here is because those with asthma are particularly concerned with the colds and flus that spread through the population during autumn and winter. Moxabustion is seen as a way of toning the body and increasing its resistance to such infection. You can either get moxa applied by a professional or use the following simple technique.

• Buy a moxa 'stick'. These are available from Chinese herb shops.

- Light the end of it and direct the burning end of the moxa stick to the *hegu* point (in the fleshy tissue between the thumb and first finger). Keep the end of the moxa stick about three to four centimetres from the *hegu* point, moving the moxa stick away and towards the point in slow motions. Remain focused or you are going to end up stabbing yourself with the hot end of the moxa stick. The inwards motion should be aimed at generating as much heat as you can comfortably tolerate. The area will start feeling warm and the texture of the skin will become oily. Allow three to five minutes on the *hegu* point of each hand.

5. POSITIVE THINKING TECHNIQUES

As previously noted the power of positive thinking should not be underestimated in its ability to develop beneficial outcomes. It is not recommended that one dispense with more traditional medical approaches but rather that one supplement these techniques with positive thinking.

When using positive thinking, always remember that it is the power of the image that you hold in your mind. You should not think about the sickness that you want to overcome or it will be the image of sickness that you hold in your mind. The image should rather be of health and energy particularly as these relate to the lungs or activities that involve the use of the lungs. The time immediately following your exercise session is an ideal opportunity for some positive imagery.

6. FENG SHUI TECHNIQUES

The Chinese art of Feng Shui operates at many levels. Basically its objective is to make the energy of the environment supportive of the energy of the individual. As such, it will deal with things as varied as making sure that the quality of the air you breathe is as beneficial as possible to looking at how the landforms, buildings, roads, and furniture that surround you influence your energy. There are obviously a number of major areas of benefit for those with asthma here. A separate publication *Feng Shui and Asthma*, available from the Academy, spells out how you might develop a Feng Shui asthma management program.

7. BODY–MIND ASPECTS OF NUTRITION

Nutrition is a very personal thing and we are not about to recommend a particular diet without knowing much more about you, personal condition and lifestyle. However, nutrition will always play an important and sometimes critical role in managing asthma and there are a number of observations that we can make that may be of use to you.

> *WARNING*
>
> *Where asthma is due to allergic response, care should be taken when trying new foods, particularly protein-based ones. Try only small amounts on the first two or three occasions and see if there is any negative response. Become a good observer of how your diet affects you and particularly what foods bring on or worsen asthma attacks. You might watch particularly for any adverse effects from dairy foods, alcohol or sugary foods.*
>
> *Where asthmatics are aspirin-sensitive, they should take medical advice in respect of the type and frequency of fish that they consume, even though a diet rich in fish would generally benefit most asthmatics.*
>
> *Where any allergen has been identified as a problem, avoid foods containing these substances. Your medical practitioner should be able to advise you as to particular foods to avoid.*

The standard approach to nutrition is to worry about what you food you buy and what food you eat but to be accurate, what should concern us is the food that is actually assimilated into the blood as macro- or micronutrients. (Macronutrients are such things as proteins, fats and carbohydrates; micronutrients are vitamins and minerals.)

When you make this change of perspective it becomes apparent that, apart from the physical constituents of the food you buy, the quantity and quality of nutrients that make it into your bloodstream will also be affected by:

- how fresh the food is when eaten;
- how well the food was stored after purchase;

- how the food was cooked;
- how the food was combined;
- how the food was presented;
- the temperature of the food at the time it was eaten;
- the environment in which the food was eaten;
- the emotional state in which the food was eaten.

From a body-mind-medicine aspect, it is the quality of energy within the food and how this is affected by the above processes that must be taken into account. As you might imagine, these issues could fill a whole book! (There is a book available from the AATC entitled *Chi Nutrition*. It deals with all the above-mentioned aspects of maintaining and enhancing the *chi* in the food we buy and maximising the body's absorption thereof.)

It is particularly important for those with asthma to ensure that the following rules are followed:

- Each meal is a relaxed, unhurried and enjoyable experience.
- Food should be well chewed before being swallowed, with attention paid to the taste and texture of the food. Sounds simple but few of us do it!
- Cold drinks with meals should be avoided as these inhibit the digestive process. Get in the habit of sipping warm water at frequent intervals. This aids the digestive process.

Dr Mark Florence and Russell Setright report in their book *Lifelong Health* that Australian research published in 1996 found that children whose diet included salmon, tuna, kingfish, mullet and trout had fewer asthma attacks. These fish are rich in selenium (see below) and N-3 fatty acids. The same source also reports that a 1994 report showed supplements of 100mg per day significantly improved lung function in asthmatics.

SOME GENERAL NOTES ON VITAMINS, MINERALS AND OTHER COMPOUNDS THAT MAY BE USEFUL IN DIET

There are a number of vitamins and minerals that have been reported as having beneficial impact on the symptoms of asthma. These include:

- vitamins A, B$_6$, C and E;
- minerals magnesium and selenium;
- sulphur and N-3 fatty acids.

Remember that cooking can destroy vitamins and that cooking in water can result in the loss of many minerals. This is particularly relevant for magnesium, which is necessary to relax the muscle cells in the bronchioles after spasm. Magnesium deficiency may also be involved in mast (hormone-producing) cell instability, causing excess histamine production, which can in turn stimulate bronchospasm.

Vitamin C is particularly important for the lungs and you should make sure your diet contains plenty of it.

ITEM	GOOD SOURCES
Vitamin A	If you're trying to increase your intake of vitamin A, *remember that this comes in two forms: • Pre-formed vitamin A from animal sources – liver, eggs, milk and butter. • Pro-vitamin A (also known as beta-carotene) from dark green leafy vegetables and yellow and orange vegetables and fruits – broccoli, kale, spinach, Brussels sprouts, apricots, cantaloupe, carrots, mangoes, papaya, peaches, squash, sweet potatoes and pumpkin. * It's unlikely that you would have any problems from a diet with too many beta-carotenes but due to dispute about the benefits/hazards of vitamin A supplements, we can only suggest caution.
Vitamin B$_6$	Pork, potatoes, spinach, 'all bran', bran flakes, muesli and avocadoes. Foods should be fresh and not overcooked.
Vitamin C	Fruits, vegetables, liver and kidneys. The best results are gained when vegetables are steamed, stir fried or microwaved. The fresher the vegetables, the more vitamin C.
Vitamin E	Vegetable oils, whole grains, peanut butter, baked sweet potatoes, avocadoes, wheatgerm, nuts (particularly almonds, peanuts and walnuts), brown rice, oatmeal, mayonnaise, margarine, corn oil and peanut oil.
Magnesium	Wheat bran, whole grains, green leafy vegetables, milk, meat beans bananas, apricots and cocoa.
Selenium	Garlic, onions, fish, shellfish, broccoli, whole wheat and grains, eggs, offal meats and chicken.
Sulphur	Garlic, broccoli, Brussels sprouts, kale and cauliflower.
Omega 3 Fatty Acids	Fish such as salmon, halibut, tuna, bass, sardines and mackerel.

Particular food items noted for having favourable impact on asthmatic conditions include:

- wild plum bark boiled in water;
- freely expressed juice of garlic mixed with honey;
- apricot and bitter apricot seed;
- steamed dried lychees;
- fresh ginger;
- ginkgo biloba;
- marshmallow;
- euphorbia.

NOTE – TAI CHI-BASED EXERCISES AND DIGESTION

Tai Chi assists digestion and thus nutrition in a number of other ways. It improves the flow of *chi* to the digestive organs, helping them to function better. It puts the body into relaxation response, which not only increases the volume of the body's resources directed to this area (blood supply for example), but also reduces the risk of gastric upset, from infection and disease within the gut (by boosting the immune system).

The gentle turning of the waist, combined with the downward pressure of the lung diaphragm in the Tai Chi breathing technique, creates a massaging effect on the intestines. This helps to keep the digestive system in trim by improving movement of food through the gut and preventing obstruction and the accumulation of putrefying material.

If you want a diet that is healthy and enjoyable – the two really do go together – you need to consider not only the quantity of what you eat and the items that make up your diet, but the way you mix your foods, how you adjust your diet to the seasons and changes in your daily activity, the quality of your food, how it is prepared, how it is presented, and how and where it is eaten.

Glossary of terms

AATC Australian Academy of Tai Chi

ABMM Program Asthma Body–Mind Medicine Program.

Acumassage use of physical pressure and manipulation on acupoints to correct *chi* energy flows.

Acupressure *see* acumassage.

Acupuncture use of needles to penetrate and stimulate acupoints to correct *chi* energy flows.

Allergy oversensitisation of the immune system to organic and inorganic chemicals.

Alveoli small sacklike structures in the lungs where the oxygen and carbon dioxide diffuses respectively into and out of the blood stream.

Assimilation absorption of nutrients from the intestines into the blood stream.

Ba Dua Gin a series of eight popular *chi kung* exercises sometimes called the eight golden treasures or the eight pieces of brocade.

Bai Hui point important acupoint used for vitality and energy. Found at the crown of the head.

Bio feedback the return of an output (such as heart rate, blood pressure, etc) as an input or stimulus with the objective of modifying the output.

Bronchi the two air passages that branch from the trachea at the base of the neck to take the air to and from each lung.

Bronchioles the air passageways that branch from each bronchi to distribute the air throughout the lungs to the alveoli.

Bronchospasm the name given to the violent inflammation and irritation of the bronchi and bronchioles that occurs during an asthma attack.

Buddha Smelling Roses name of *chi kung* movement used in the supplementary exercises of the ABMM program.

Chan San Feng legendary creator of Tai Chi.

Chi the name given to the vital energy that drives all activity in the universe.

Chi breathing breathing techniques that focus on the extraction of *chi* from the air.

Chi diet a form of diet where the focus is on the quantity, nature and quality of the *chi* that is obtained from one's diet.

Chi kung literally 'skill with energy'.

Chi meditation use of mental focus to encourage the proper flow of *chi* throughout the body.

Chen-style Tai Chi the first historical form of Tai Chi. A fairly vigorous martial arts-based Tai Chi.

Chi hai point important acupoint three finger-widths below the navel. Involved with the extraction of *chi* from the breathing process.

Cleansing Breath breathing technique detailed in Part 4 that is particularly useful for smokers or clearing polluted air from the lungs.

Colon another name for the large intestine. Functions are retention of water and elimination.

Conception vessel Another name for the *ren mai* – the extraordinary meridian that runs down the front centre of the body torso.

Dao Yin Chinese exercise system developed more than 2500 years ago that focused on breathing, posture and energy circulation. Sometimes called *Tao Yin*.

Diaphragmatic breathing breathing that is primarily driven on the in-breath by the downward movement of the lung diaphragm and on the out-breath by the upward movement of the lung diaphragm.

Digestion the body's process of breaking down complex nutrients into simpler nutrients in the digestive tract.

Du Mo meridian *see* governing vessel.

Eight Golden Treasures *see Ba Dua Gin*.

Endocrine glands glands that secrete hormones that modify metabolic and growth activity within the body.

Extraordinary meridians name given to the eight meridians that deal with the balancing of energy within the body.

Five Elements theory the theory that deals with the five elemental energy phases of *chi* – wood, fire, earth, metal, water.

Genetic predisposition the increased likelihood of developing a particular condition because of one's genetic heritage.

Governing vessel another name for the *du mo* meridian that runs up the centre of the back, over the head and down the centre front of the head.

Heavenly Lift one of the *Ba Dua Gin* exercises used in the ABMM program.

Hegu point important acupoint used for vitality and energy. Found in the fleshy tissue between the thumb and first finger.

Horse-riding stance an important training stance with straight back, bent knees and the sensation of gripping a horse with the legs.

Hsueh the Chinese name for acupoint, which more correctly describes the area as a cavern of *chi*.

Immune function/system the body's systems that deal with defence against infection and injury.

Ingestion the process of taking food into the body.

Intercoastal muscles the muscles that expand the upper rib cage and are used in chest breathing.

Inhaler device for getting a chemical vapour to the lungs that helps inhibit the bronchospasm process.

Khor-style Tai Chi Grandmaster Khor's version of the large frame Yang-style Tai Chi, fine-tuned for health and relaxation.

Lao Gong point Important acupoint at the centre of the palm.

Large intestine *see* colon.

Large intestine meridian the energy meridian that is paired with the lung meridian and thus has particular importance to asthmatics.

Lesser Heavenly circulation the energy circulation pathway that is formed by the *du mo* and *ren mai* meridians.

Lotus body-toning relaxation system *chi kung* exercise system used at AATC.

Lung capacity vital the total volume of air that the lungs can take in on a single breath.

Lung capacity effective the total volume that is actually taken in on a full in-breath due to postural and muscular problems. Will always be less than the vital capacity.

Lung diaphragm the sheet of muscle that separates the chest and abdominal cavity, and is used in diaphragmatic breathing.

Lung membrane the tissue that forms the walls of the alveoli.

Lymph the fluid that is circulated through the body and lymphatic system.

Lymphatic system the system that generates and filters the lymph fluid that has much to do with the control of infection.

Medical practitioner means primary health consultant, including registered medical practitioner or other health consultants if you have chosen a practitioner from the alternative health care area.

Meng mun a very important acupoint on the spine opposite the navel.

Meridian energy channel that carries *chi*.

Mian silk-like movement. Movement without jerkiness or abrupt changes of direction.

Moxabustion burning of moxa herbs over acupoints to stimulate energy flow.

Nasal breathing in-breath and out-breath through the nose.

Organ meridian energy channel that supports an organ function.

Osteoporosis loss of calcium from bones which results in increased risk of breakage and fracture.

Oxygen debt the drop of oxygen levels in the blood due to sudden vigorous exercise.

PNI *see* psychoneuroimmunology.

Positive thinking various mental techniques that use positive imagery and affirmation within thought.

Psychoneuroimmunology the science that looks at the connection between mental states and the operation of the immune system.

Reflexology the recognition that the body has a holistic nature and that various parts of the body may have relationships to other parts (often far removed). Massage or manipulation of these 'reflex zones or points' can be used to influence the functioning of the connected point.

Ren Mai meridian *see* conception vessel.

Respiratory system the system that deals with the taking in of oxygen and the release of carbon dioxide from the body.

Shen spirit in the sense of being high-spirited. State of the emotional energy and feeling of well-being.

Shibashi series of 18 Tai Chi *chi kung* exercises – popular in China and taught by the AATC as an introductory Tai Chi *chi kung*.

Silk-like movement *see* Mian.

Su Liao point acupoint at tip of nose that is involved in breathing.

Tai Chi often used as an abbreviation for Tai Chi Chuan (literally the supreme ultimate fist), also used to describe any exercise that contains the principles outlined in the Tai Chi Ching. Principles involve relaxation, breathing, posture, slow movement, *mian*, *chi kung* techniques, martial arts applications.

Tai Chi breathing breathing that involves unforced diaphragmatic breathing with inhalation and exhalation through the nose.

Tai Chi Ching classic writings on Tai Chi by masters such as Chan San Feng.

Tai Chi massage massage techniques that focus on relaxation, the flow of *chi*, and posture.

Tai Chi stretching stretching that involves using muscles against each other rather than against the joints. Thus there is never a full extension of the limbs; rather one extends the limb as simultaneously pulling back.

Tao literally 'the way' that the universe operates and evolves. Sometimes called the 'dao'.

Tao Yin *see* dao yin.

Taoist a follower of the Tao.

Taoist Archer a movement from the *Ba Dua Gin* used in the ABMM program.

Tan Tien the area in front of and between the kidneys. The area in the body which stores *chi*.

Tidal volume the total volume of the air breathed in over a given period of time.

Trachea the large airway that runs from the pharynx to the two bronchi.

Turbelles structures in the nose that disrupt the flow of air in a manner that allows the nasal surface to increase its contact with the air being breathed in, increasing the efficiency of the filtration. It is a heating and moistening process.

Venous blood return system the system of veins, venous valves and muscles that acts to pump the blood back towards the heart as the limbs are moved during physical activity.

Wei Chi the defensive energy that surrounds the body like an envelope preventing infection. In Chinese terms, bacteria and viruses survive to infect the body when the *wei chi* is weak.

Yang the positive active nature of *chi*.

Yang-style Tai Chi the Tai Chi form devised by the Yang family.

Yin the passive, gathering nature of *chi*.

Yin–Yang theory the theory that *chi* has two basic natures, yin and yang, which need to be balanced and harmonised.

Yun men chief lung meridian acupoint.

Appendix 1

About Tai Chi

There are many forms or styles of Tai Chi such as *yang, sun, chen, wu* and *ho* to name but a few. What makes these all these exercises Tai Chi is adherence to the principles espoused in the *Tai Chi Ching Classics* (a record of what the leading Tai Chi masters considered important about Tai Chi). While these principles are generally learned through the practice of forms (connected sequences of movements that may be up to 108 movements long), the principles can be equally applied to any activity from exercise to massage.

The practice of Tai Chi exercise forms has long been acknowledged as a safe and enjoyable way of maintaining and improving overall health. This is due to the fact that the exercises are focused on 'health' rather than 'fitness'. Fitness focuses you on what you can 'do' as opposed to what your exercise is 'doing' to you. It is concerned with such things as:

- how fast and how far can you run?
- how high can you jump?

- how many push-ups or chin-ups can you do?
- how much weight can you lift?

Thus if you can run a long distance, you are fit despite the fact that what you are doing is causing your knees and spine to deteriorate and will result in pain and reduced mobility in later years. On the other hand, when you do a health exercise, the focus is always on improving your long-term health and quality of life. After several thousand years of experimenting with exercises for health (the Chinese have recorded that the first 'government'-prescribed health exercise program was initiated by the Emperor Huang Di around 2800BC he prescribed a series of health dances 'for the population to perform'), the Chinese decided that exercises based on a combination of posture, 'silk-like' movement, diaphragmatic breathing, body–mind integration and awareness were the most effective way of developing long-term health. Since these are the five principles that underly Tai Chi, I refer to any exercise that embodies all these principles as a Tai Chi-based exercise.

With the focus of Tai Chi-based exercises on relaxation and breathing techniques, it would seem only natural that the practice of such exercises would help improve the health of people with breathing-related disorders such as asthma. Indeed, as noted in Part 1, the main factor that stimulated the creation of this program was the many positive comments received from asthmatic students attending our standard courses.

Appendix 2

How the ABMM Program Developed

In my role as Grandmaster of the Australian Academy of Tai Chi, I have overseen an organisation that has trained more than 100,000 students in various Chinese exercise systems. As such, I have had constant feedback from students as to how the exercise courses taught by the Academy have impacted on their lives and health.

I began to notice that many students had asthma but were reporting favourable outcomes in the improvement of their condition after becoming involved with Academy courses. Such comments included:

- reduction in frequency and severity of attacks;
- reduced requirement for medication;
- increased sense of vitality and energy; and
- increased stamina and strength.

Being aware that Academy courses are not specifically focused towards asthma, I began to wonder whether or not people with asthma could not benefit even further if their attention was directed to the particular elements of Academy courses that would be of particular benefit. On the one hand, I did not want to give these students the impression that they should not remain part of the mainstream. On the other hand, I recognised that a program that focused on key techniques and exercises that were particularly useful for asthmatics could bring benefits more quickly than our normal student courses. These are, of necessity, more general in application and revolve around the teaching of the Tai Chi form (which can take two years to become proficient in). Additionally, valuable techniques for asthma students such as acumassage and *chi* visualisation might not be encountered for some time by a student going through our standard program of courses. My solution was to produce a booklet titled 'Managing Asthma with *Chi* Exercise' and make this available to students within Academy classes. The program was designed to be used in the following ways.

- Firstly, it could be used to enhance existing Academy courses. Students with asthma would learn to understand more about how the exercises they were learning in class could work for them and bias their own practice to the exercises with the greatest benefit for their condition.
- Secondly, the booklet was structured in such a manner that non-Academy students could learn and practise their own 'model lesson' specifically related to managing asthma. I felt that this was particularly important because of the number of children who were developing asthma. The program was easy to learn and could be mastered in days

All the techniques and exercises used in the program are simple enough to be learned and practised by the ordinary person (though supervision by parents will be appropriate in the case of young children). Since the focus was asthma rather than health through exercise, I increased the techniques available to include acumassage, diet and aromatherapy aspects from the Academy's 'Living Chi' program to supplement the postural, movement, breathing and positive visualisation techniques extracted from course material. The booklet was well received and there was obviously a much larger need for such a program than could be filled through an 'in-house' booklet. To meet this need, I added considerably more detail and information on asthma and how it works to the material contained within the booklet. The final result is this book. The ABMM program is still designed to be used the same way, either as an enhancement to classes for existing students with an asthma condition or as a stand-alone program for those who cannot or choose not to attend one of the Academy's regular instructor-led classes.

Appendix 3

Resources

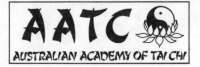

The further resources that are available from AATC to supplement or further develop the material provided in this book are listed below.

SPECIFIC EXERCISES

- Quiet Standing – the starting position of the Tai Chi set. See *Tai Chi Level 1–3* book and *Tai Chi Level 1* on video.

- Shoulder-rolling exercises – one of the joint relaxation techniques used as warm-up exercises for Tai Chi. See *Joint Exercise* booklet for full joint exercise program.

- Swinging arms exercise – one of the eight golden treasures exercises used to accompany the Tai Chi courses. See *Eight Golden Treasures* booklet. Heavenly Lift and Taoist Archer also come from this booklet.

- Abdominal Massage – taken from acupressure massage work-shops. See Acupressure booklets 1 (Head, neck and shoulders), 2 (Hands), 3 (Feet), 4 (Abdominal Massage). Lung meridian work also comes from here.

- Breathing Visualisations – taken from *Chi Breathing* booklet and workshop.

- Opening the Chest exercise – the second exercise of the Shibashi Tai Chi Qi Qong sequence from the book *Tai Chi Qi Qong* for *Stress Control and Relaxation*. Also the video of same name.

GENERAL RESOURCES RELATED TO ABOVE MATERIAL

- History and Philosophy of Tai Chi booklet.
- *Chi* Diet and Nutrition booklet
- Dynamic Relaxation booklet
- Relaxing music tapes

STATE OFFICES

New South Wales
(National Head Office)
PO Box 1020
Burwood North NSW 2134
Tel/Fax: (02) 9797 9355

Queensland
PO Box 2475
Fortitude Valley QLD 4006
Tel: (07) 3358 1955

South Australia
GPO Box 1306
Adelaide SA 5001
Tel: (08) 8287 3571

Western Australia
7 Crofton Place
Lynwood WA 7147
Tel: (08) 9258 3434
e-mail: westchi@iprimus.com.au

Tasmania
Tel: (03) 6393 6963

The AATC is happy to assist in enquiries in respect of acquisition of the above materials and can be contacted at:

Website: www.livingchi.com.au
e-mail: livinchi@ihug.com.au

REGIONAL OFFICES

New South Wales
Albury/Corowra (02) 6033 3172
Baradine (02) 6843 1982
Central Coast (02) 4332 7176
Coonabarabran (02) 6842 2079
Kootingal (02) 6765 8292
Newcastle (02) 4942 2951
Orange (02) 6565 8309
Tamworth (02) 6765 8292
Wollongong (02) 4261 5786

Queensland
Bundaberg (07) 4153 4428
Gold Coast (07) 5572 8921
Gympie (07) 5486 5131
Rockhampton (07) 4939 5845
Sunshine Coast (07) 5491 2314
Toowoomba (07) 4636 5034

EDUCATION SERVICES

Standard courses: Community classes are held in most areas. Private instruction also available.

Seminars and workshops are also held regularly in main centres. Grandmaster Khor and others are also available to come to your areas to present a workshop or seminar.

Corporate, children's and seniors' packages can be tailored to your needs.

Talks and demonstrations. including guest speakers, can be arranged.

Instructor training courses and business franchises are available.

HOME LEARNING AND COURSE BACK-UP

Videos
Tai Chi for Health and Relaxation
Stress Control the Eastern Way
Qigong Shibashi: The 18 Techniques
Khor Tai Chi: Moving Meditation
Wellness Exercise: Lotus, Lohan and Sword

Books by Grandmaster Gary Khor
Tai Chi for Stress Control and Relaxation
Feng Shui for Personal Harmony: Enhancing Your Life with the Ancient Art of Placement
Living Chi: The Ancient Chinese Way to Bring Life Energy and Harmony into Your Life

Music Tapes
Exclusive oriental music for Tai Chi and Qigong exercises.
Also excellent for meditation, relaxation, background music, or just easy listening.

'Beginnings' – peaceful and relaxing
'Tao Yin' – oriental bamboo flute and string music
'Lohan' – beautiful Qigong music
'Tai Chi' music for relaxation

Bibliography

Attack Asthma – William Vayda. ISBN 0-85091-626-7

A Parents Guide to Allergies and Asthma, Marion Steinmann, Dell
Publishing. ISBN 0-385-30029-8

Understanding Asthma, Maria Prendergast, The Text Publishing Company
Melbourne Australia. ISBN 1-86372-025-1

Breathing Easy – A parents' guide to dealing with your child's asthma,
Maryanne Stevens, Prentice Hall Press. ISBN 0-13-083692-3

Give Asthma the Big A, Marian Shepherd Lee, Bookman Press. ISBN 1-
86395-152-0

Freedom from Asthma, Alexander Stalmatski, Hale Clinic Health Library.
ISBN 1-85626-268-5

Asthma the facts, Donald J. Lane. ISBN 0-19-262151-3

Oriental Breathing Therapy, Takashi Nakamura, Japan Publications Inc.
ISBN 0-87040-478-4

The Ear – Gateway to balancing the body – Mario Wexu D. Ac. ISBN: 0-
88231-022-4

Finger Acupressure, Dr P C Chan. Published Life and Health Centre Ltd
Hong Kong 1990.

Reflexology, Inge Dougans. The Bridgewater Book Company. ISBN 1-
85230-874-5.

Acupuncture Medicine, Yoshiaki Omura Sc.D, M.D. Japan Publications Inc.
ISBN 0-87040-491-1

Anatomical Atlas of Chinese Acupuncture points, Published Shandong
Science and Technology Press. 1982

Eating Your Way to Health, Dietotherapy in Traditional Chinese Medicine
Cai Jin Feng. Foreign Languages Press Beijing. ISBN 0-8351-1953-X

Chinese System of Food Cures, Henry C Lu, Sterling Publishing Company New York. ISBN 0-8069-6308-5

Food as Medicine. Earl Mindell R.Ph. Ph.D., Bookman Press Melbourne. ISBN 1-86395-061-3

Chinese Tonic Herbs, Ron Teeguarden, Japan Publications Inc. ISBN 0-87040-551-9

Secrets of the Chinese Herbalists, Richard Lucas, Parker Publishing Company, New York. ISBN 0-13-797621-6

Aromatherapy, a Holistic Guide, Ann Berwick. Llewellyn Publications USA. ISBN 0-87542-033-8

Aromatherapy and Natural Health Magazine, Issue 1

Lifelong Health, Dr Mark Florence and Russell Setright, Hodder and Stoughton

Mind–body Medicine, edited Daniel Goleman, Ph.D. and Joel Gurin. ISBN 0-947277-18-8

Living Chi, Grandmaster Gary Khor. Simon and Schuster Australia, East Roseville, Sydney. ISBN 0-7318-0757-X

Tai Chi for Stress Control, Grandmaster Gary Khor, Simon and Schuster Australia, East Roseville, Sydney. ISBN 0-7318-0361-2

Tai Chi for a Healthy Lifestyle, Grandmaster Gary Khor, New Holland, Sydney. ISBN 186436574-9

Index